Contents

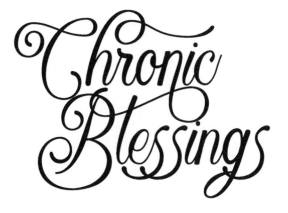

Chronic Blessings

Finding Life's Greatest Joys Within Your Deepest Heartache

Cristy Maddox

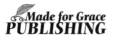

Made for Grace
PUBLISHING

COLUMBIA

MAY 2 4 2019

Made for Grace Publishing
P.O. Box 1775 Issaquah, WA 98027

Designed by DeeDee Heathman
Editor: Katie Rios
Executive Editor: Valerie Heathman
Author Photo Credit: Peyton Farmer

Library of Congress Cataloging-in-Publication data
Maddox, Cristy.
Chronic Blessings: Finding Life's Greatest Joys within
Your Deepest Heartache
p. cm.
ISBN: 978-1-64146-354-6 (pbk.)
ISBN: 978-1-64146-362-1 (eBook)
LCCN: 2018956065

To contact the publisher please email Service@MadeForSuccess.net or
call +1 425 657 0300.

Made for Grace Publishing is an imprint of Made for Success, inc.
Printed in the United States of America

DEDICATION

Greg,

You have had to learn the true meaning of "for better, for worse; in sickness and in health" far too young. Not only have you proven yourself to be a man of your word, but even in the midst of all the chaos, you still manage to encourage, support and empower me to chase my ridiculous dreams. Thank you for loving me and believing that God will come through.

You forever have my love and gratitude.

Introduction

As I sit clinging to my purse in the icebox otherwise known as the Detroit Metro Airport, I have learned to set much of my pride aside for my own safety. I've had no choice. There are so many lessons I have had to learn the hard way, one of which I've just implemented: asking for help.

However, as I sit here alone while the minutes tick by, I'm not sure if the help is coming. I'm not even sure if the woman at the counter understood what I was saying.

I know that it is hard to understand me when my speech becomes slurred, and the panic that was starting to set in probably didn't help either. But I hope that she at least got the message that I need help. She told me to sit to the side and wait.

So, I'm waiting. It's not as if I have any other choice.

The terminal is now empty; all the other passengers have returned home or gone to find hotels. I just wish I knew what to do. As I begin to feel more and more alone, I can't help but wonder: If I were 80 and walked with a cane, would I have been left here for this long?

And I can't believe that this is actually happening. *This* is why I was so afraid to make this trip alone. Yet, I had been doing so well that I kind of felt like I was being a big baby about it. The flight out was perfect, and the days with my publisher went beautifully. I was excited to share about what God has done in my life, and the innumerable lessons I've learned. My confidence was renewed, and even though I was totally exhausted from the trip, I wasn't the slightest bit worried about the return flights home.

Sure, my heart rate was sky-high and my right leg was starting to feel a little weak, but I expected those things to be happening after the busy days I just had—especially considering I just had to stand in line for an hour to get through security. In fact, I would have been shocked if those things *didn't* happen.

Even though I felt pretty bad after the security line, I made it from Seattle to Detroit in one piece. I even made it on and off the train from one terminal to the next and walked through a crazy tunnel with flashing disco lights—without losing my balance or getting sick. Overall, I thought I was doing pretty well.

But then the delays started; one after another until it was after 10 p.m. When another delay was announced, I got up to use the restroom. Unfortunately, my right knee started to buckle on the way. Not a good sign. It's sort of like the rumble of thunder just before the downpour. If you can run back inside, you'll be safe from the rain, wind and lightning.

But I had nowhere to run. I *needed* to get on that plane.

As I made my way back to my gate, the noise and light began to intensify. I decided to sit at another empty gate that was far enough away to be quiet, but close enough that I could still hear the announcements. It seemed like a good plan at the time. However, when they announced that the flight had been postponed until noon the next day, I was too far away and too slow to make it to the counter before everyone else was already in line.

I managed to text Greg with the new flight info, but I was in bad shape by this point—dizzy, weak, blurred vision and having a hard time bearing weight on my right leg. And then the long wait in line; that was the final straw that did me in.

When I reached the front of the line, all I could do was lean on the counter and say, "I need help." The woman was busy printing my new ticket for the next day. "What do you need help with?"

I couldn't think. I could barely stand. I didn't know what to say, so I muttered, "I need ... I just ... don't know what to do. Can't stand."

The lady told me to go sit to the side, and she would call someone.

That was an hour ago. It is quiet, and I am sitting with my legs up on the metal chairs. I keep looking at my phone—there are multiple missed messages from Greg. I know I could use my phone to help me figure out something, but I just don't know what ... or how. As I stare at my phone realizing just how incapable I am, the tears start to trickle down my face. And then they pour.

I am all-out sobbing when a woman walks up to see what I need. I do my best to pull myself together. The woman explains that the airline is not covering hotels due to this being a weather-related delay, but that they can give me a discount voucher.

"What do I do with that?"

"You decide on what hotel you'd like to stay at, call and book your hotel and then take one of our shuttles directly to the hotel."

She may as well have told me to build my own airplane and fly it home.

I look down at my phone and think a minute. Realizing I can't do any of the things she is telling me to do, I simply reply through my tears, "I can't do that."

"You can't?"

"I ... don't know how. I don't think I can walk." At least I'm making a little sense.

"Well, we can have someone take you to where you get your discount voucher. Then, once you book your hotel, they can take you to the shuttle."

It still sounds like rocket science to me. I look down at my phone again and the multiple missed messages from Greg. The wheels are turning. I just know there must be some simple solution ... but it is over my head. "I can't."

"Well ... you can stay here."

Now I'm crying harder.

"I can get someone to take you to a place in the airport that has chairs that are a little more comfortable. We will get you a blanket and a pillow."

"Okay."

She disappears, and my crying continues. I know a night in the airport will be miserable. But that's not the reason for my tears. I'm crying because of how utterly helpless and pathetic I feel. I'm an adult who can't figure out how to book a hotel! I'm an adult who can't figure out how to use my phone to let my husband know what's going on! And I'm crying because I know this is going to set me back physically.

I'm still sobbing when a man comes with a wheelchair and starts to load up my carry-on bags. As he pushes me through the airport, I rest my chin on the bags on my lap, and despite all my attempts to stop, I am still bawling my eyes out. It is after midnight, and the airport is quiet. I have never felt so alone.

In that exact moment, I distinctly hear God say, "It's time to put your money where your mouth is. Am I truly enough?"

At first, I cry harder because it felt like a knife to the heart. I'm thinking, *You've got to be kidding me! I'm really supposed to learn some lesson ... right now?! That's too much to expect. I don't even have half a brain cell.* But I suck in my sobs and say to Him, "What a crappy way to extend this lesson, God! My head knows that you are enough, but my heart ... not so much right now. But, yes; I believe you are enough. Please show me that fact tonight. I don't know how I'm going to get through this. This could totally do me in. Help me get through this."

"Here we are," the man says softly as he finds me the crème de la crème of airport chairs within 10 feet of a restroom. He gives me a pillow, two blankets and leaves the wheelchair with me so my belongings can be safely tucked underneath.

My pathetic brain remembers that I need my medication, that I have a sleep aid and that I have earplugs. I pull my coat hoodie over my head to block out the light, and I get the best airport-night's-sleep in the history of the Detroit Metro.

Chapter One

According to Plan

*"Many are the plans in the mind of a man, but it
is the purpose of the Lord that will stand."*
— Proverbs 19:21, ESV

Even as a child, I loved the sense of accomplishment I felt
after a lot of hard work. There were days that I was too
busy to play; but believe it or not, I genuinely enjoyed
those times. I felt proud of being responsible for many things.

Conveniently, that came with the territory as we were a busy
family, living in the country with a lot to do. I have two older sisters
and a younger brother, as well as another girl who I will always
consider a sister because she lived with us for years. Besides work
around the house, we kept busy helping in the garden, working on
my grandpa's farm or cleaning houses with my mother.

When there wasn't work to be done, there was plenty of fun to
be had; go-carts, scooters, building forts in the woods, swimming
in my grandpa's bowl-shaped pool in the summer and riding bikes
in it during the winter. With my grandparents living on one side
of us and my great aunt and uncle on the other side, we had plenty
of land to roam.

When I was 12, my sisters were away staying with relatives due to poor schooling options in our area, and my mother became sick with Lyme disease. I hated that my mom was suffering, and she hated that so much of the burden of the household fell on me. But I didn't mind the responsibility. The feeling of being needed was something that gave me joy, and I gained a lot of satisfaction when I was able to prove to my family that they could depend on me. Because I have a caretaker personality, I found that I enjoyed this feeling more than the fun of play.

Maybe that's why I dreamed so much about children. Marriage was definitely important to me, but what I thought about most was taking care of my children. I wanted three to five kids, and I wanted at least one of them to come to me through adoption. To me, the thought of having a family without adoption in the picture was something I couldn't fathom. Two of my mom's brothers, my dad's sister and one of my own sisters were all adopted. Having been raised with such a beautiful culture of adoption, it simply seemed like a natural part of having a family.

I did dream of having a good job, but it was more important to me that the job would be able to take a backseat to raising my kids. As I entered college, I dreamed of living overseas as a missionary—not necessarily long term, but for a couple of years at least. I wanted to take my kids on mission trips and open their eyes to the world around them. I longed for them to live lives of service with an outward focus, like Jesus did.

It all seemed so simple then, but maybe that was me being one of those annoying, make-you-want-to-gag kind of people who had a pretty easy, uncomplicated life. I had the best parents ever, and amazing siblings; I even had four incredible, healthy grandparents.

Of course, my family and I went through difficult times, but overall, I had it good—so stinkin' good. I planned everything out, and everything went according to my plan. Decisions came easily to my clear, focused mind.

By my senior year of high school, I knew exactly what career I wanted. I began working toward that goal the summer before college actually started—no time, class, or money wasted. College was a blast, not only because I got good grades and had great friends, but also because I received scholarships for working with campus ministries and playing women's fast pitch softball.

My first day of college, I met the love of my life, whom I have now been married to for 20 years. Greg was—and is—God's perfect match for me, and I didn't even have to wait for him. He is the kind of guy who makes me laugh, even when I don't want to. He is easygoing enough to go with the flow of my type A agenda, yet not *too* laid back that he drives my type A personality mad.

He was totally on board with my very clear goals in life, and even though we were practically babies when we got married (20 and 21), we stuck to those goals. Just days after my 23rd birthday, I graduated with my masters in physical therapy, and two years later he finished college as a physician assistant. We were living in Ohio, and we had purchased the most adorable little house I have ever seen. We had incredible friends surrounding us. Life was good.

Sickening, isn't it? Easy. Too easy actually. When everything in life is a piece of cake, and all is well around us, we tend to keep our eyes on the things of the world. What we truly need is to be looking *up*. When we don't look up—or don't look up enough—God loves us enough to allow us to fall so low that we don't like what we see on our own level. Eventually, when we get sick of crawling around in the mud, we will look up to see if there is something better.

When my vision becomes too horizontal, I am grateful for a God who loves me enough to give me mud.

—∞—

A couple years after Greg and I were married, we were part of a weekly Bible study and prayer group with a few friends. We were blessed with amazing men and women in our lives who had very deep connections with God. You would think being surrounded by people like that would have strengthened one's faith. Oddly enough, it seemed to weaken mine. Because of their deep relationships, these friends often shared stories of God's presence and the way He spoke to them. They were beautiful stories.

And they made me mad.

Why was God talking to everyone else but me? I felt like I was pursuing God. I was going to church, praying and meeting for these Bible studies. So ... what was the holdup? Why didn't I get to experience God the same way that my friends were?

I struggled with this for a long time, and began to have a crisis of faith. I called out to God and did not receive answers. At the time, I could not understand it. Why was God so utterly silent?

Looking back, I am now convinced that He didn't speak because I did not sincerely see my need for Him. All was going smoothly, and I was so self-sufficient. I needed these friends and their maddening, sickeningly sweet stories of their talks with God to clue me in to what I was missing. I needed His silence—combined with examples of what a relationship with Him could look like—to make me truly seek to know Him personally.

I continued to struggle with His silence. At one of my lowest points in this journey, we went with a group from our church to Willow Creek, a megachurch in a northwest Chicago suburb that was founded by Bill Hybels. They were having a youth leaders' training session, and for some reason (that is totally beyond me now), I thought I'd be interested in working with youth. The music and worship atmosphere there was powerful, and I was swept up in the experience. I felt alive because I could feel God's presence in that church and in myself. It was a spiritual high point. I was grateful—and also relieved—that God had once again made Himself known to me.

However, by the next weekend, when we were back at our own church, I felt dead again. Dead and angry. Angry at God, and angry at *myself.* Why did I need some big production in order to feel His presence? And had it even been His presence in the first place if I could no longer feel Him?

I found myself sitting in a bathroom stall, staring at the walls for what seemed like forever. I began yelling at God, "Where are you? Why have you left me alone?" In an attempt to pull myself together, I'd walk out of the bathroom, only to start crying again and run back in. Each time I'd endeavor to exit the bathroom, Greg would say, "Let's just go home."

But I couldn't. I was desperate. I wanted to stay ... I *needed* to stay.

Eventually, I pulled myself together and walked into the sanctuary. The sermon had already started, and we sat down in the back. I listened with rapt attention as the pastor continued ...

"Such a dark, cold, lonely pit. How long did Joseph stare at those walls and cry out to God, 'Where are you? Why have you left me alone?'"

Chills ran down my spine as I recognized those exact words. Pulling myself together had been pointless because now I was bawling all over again.

Poor Joseph had been thrown in that pit by his brothers and was about to be sold into slavery and taken to Egypt.

How could I compare that to my life?! I was nowhere near Joseph's desperate situation, but I sure could relate to how he felt in that pit. I thought God had left me alone.

Joseph likely thought the same, but God had incredible plans for Joseph. He would be second in command of Egypt. He would save his family, his people and the Egyptians from starvation. Sure, he was also going to be ripped away from his family, forced into slavery, accused of rape and imprisoned for years. It would not be easy, to say the least. I'm sure it was not what Joseph dreamed of when he planned his future, but I doubt at the end of his life that he would have had it any other way. He would consider all of the trials and pain he had endured as worth the cost.

Looking at Joseph's life, it felt a bit silly to have been so upset over God's silence. Yet I was still relieved that He had chosen to make Himself known to me through Joseph's story. It is hard to truly convey the power of that moment and how it renewed my faith.

I was now able to recognize God's presence more frequently—without the need for a big Willow Creek production. Life was still pretty good, and since the crisis of faith had passed, I slipped back into my normal routine.

Although from the outside my normal routine looked, well, normal, on the inside it was anything but. When I was at home, I was worrying about what I needed to do at work. When I was at work, I was worrying about what I needed to do at home. My schedule spun in my head like a hamster on a wheel. Always planning, always scheduling. How could I fit the most into my day? Get the most done?

There was always so much to do, and I didn't even have kids yet! I was working in home health as a physical therapist, so there were work calls and scheduling to be done at home. But it wouldn't have mattered if I had worked in a different setting; I let everything consume me, consume my mind.

When I managed to take the time to sit and try to pray or read, the hamster kept running. I could not make him stop. My house was always clean, and laundry could not possibly pile up. Spider webs beware!

But, I thought this was normal. I thought every woman was like this. After all, we had our young adult group from our church over to our house a couple times a month, and friends over much more often than that. So, the house *had* to be clean, right? Still, it was a good thing that we had friends around so much, because enjoying the company of other people was the best thing I could do to slow the hamster's pace.

I knew that my constant planning and analyzing behaviors were annoying. Honestly, I truly wished that I could just let things go and chill. But I did not recognize it for what it really was, and I don't think I ever would have if life had continued on its smooth, neatly charted path.

—∞∞—

Next up on my clearly planned life timeline was to have a baby. I was so ready. We had married young and had a lot of school to get through first, so it felt like we had already waited forever. Greg was nearing the completion of physician assistant school, so we were in the clear, time-wise. We could start trying for a baby, and if it happened right away, school would be finished by the time the baby came. He would start working, and I would cut back to part-time.

But as each month came and went, my plan began to crumble. I would chart everything out so carefully; when my period started, I'd cry my eyes out, then try to encourage myself by figuring out what the next due date would be *if* it happened that month. That new date would become my new goal, and I'd start planning everything around it in my mind. Each month I didn't become pregnant, I was more and more devastated. Most sensible-minded women would give it at least a year, but I was so anxious that I scheduled an appointment with my obstetrician about nine months into the process.

When I told my doc the situation, she gave me a grid to map my temperature first thing each morning. According to how my temperature changed, I should be able to tell when I ovulated.

Sweet! That should help.

But the temperatures told me nothing. I even bought some expensive ovulation testing kits to pee on every single day. Nothing. So, back to the doctor I went. She decided to do further testing and discovered that I wasn't ovulating at all.

I couldn't have been more terrified. She put me on a medication that would help me ovulate, and I was to return on a specific day of my cycle for lab work. The first month showed no change, so, she increased the dose. The second month came and went, still no change. She increased the dose again, but this time informed me that this was as high as we could go. If it didn't work this time, then we would have to pursue a fertility specialist.

Throughout this process, I prayed more than I had probably prayed in my previous 25 years combined. I begged and I pleaded, then I pleaded and begged some more. I was so hopeful that each method or dose would work. After all, I was doing everything I possibly could to help the situation along.

With each failed month, I became increasingly more discouraged. I was anxious and stressed. I didn't know what else to do! I was researching and doing everything within *my* power, including natural cleanses, eating healthy and doing everything my doctor told me—to a "T."

As I was pleading with God one morning, I suddenly heard Him say, "Don't you think I know?"

It stopped me in my tracks. Well, of course He knew.

"Then don't you think you could trust Me with this?"

I thought about it, and yes, *of course* I should trust Him with it. That should have been obvious to me. But that tug on my heart to take control was overwhelming.

"But God, I just don't know what to do."

"Then don't *do* anything."

Believe it or not, that was the hardest thing He could have asked. But, as hardheaded as I was, the more I thought about it, the more I fully understood what God was really telling me. He was saying, "You've got to get a grip. And by getting a grip, I mean, you've got to let go. You try to control every detail of your life, and that just isn't going to serve you well. You may be able to control a few things in life, but you won't be able to control the things that truly matter. This is your chance to learn to surrender something of true importance to you and show Me that you really do trust Me."

It was a light bulb moment. A realization that God was trying to teach me something through this heartbreaking situation. A realization that my hardships could have a profound purpose and contain more meaning than just what was visible on the surface. A realization that, in every circumstance, there truly is more than meets the eye.

So, I took a deep breath and said it: "Okay God. I will trust You with this. You know how desperately we want this. You ultimately know what is best, so I'm leaving it in Your hands. But You've got to help me leave it there. Remind me not to try to take it back from You every few minutes!" Then I took a step back and instead of feeling freaked out at my lack of ability to *do* something, I felt much more at peace about it. Relieved, as a matter of fact.

When I went in for my lab work, they told me, "If you don't hear anything, then it's good news. We will call you if there is a problem and we need to discuss the next steps." The next two days dragged on and on. Every time the phone rang, I cringed and then let out a sigh of relief when the voice on the other end was not from my doctor's office.

Then I got the call. "Crystal, I am calling to let you know about your lab work."

Tears immediately sprung into my eyes, and a massive lump filled my throat.

"Everything looks good. It looks like this dose worked, and you are ovulating. The doctor says we will just keep you at this dose, and hopefully something will happen for you soon."

Now the tears were really falling, but they were tears of joy. Apparently, someone hadn't gotten the message not to call if all looked good.

Three months later, at 5 a.m. on a Sunday, I peed on a stick. Greg has never woken up to a louder squeal of joy.

———◦⧟◦———

As soon as Aiden was born, we realized how important it was to us to be near family again and began working toward returning to Virginia to be near both sets of our parents. It was particularly hard for us to leave our friends in Ohio, but family was a huge draw for us, so we moved back when Aiden was about two years old. I was pregnant with our second son, Noah, at the time. We bought a house in the country 10 minutes down the road from my parents, and only 40 minutes from my in-laws.

We both had good jobs. I was working in a local hospital every Monday and two Sundays a month which was perfect to support our finances, get me around some adult conversation and keep one foot in the physical therapy field.

We were thrilled with where we were. I had always wanted to live in the country, and God had worked an amazing miracle with our house in Ohio. At the exact same moment that we made an offer on our house in Virginia, an offer was placed on our house in Ohio. We felt confident that we were exactly where He wanted us.

Things were going smoothly with the boys, and I finally felt ready to pursue some of the things that God had placed on my heart.

I had a passion for service and became a volunteer for Compassion International. We had sponsored a child with Compassion since our first year of marriage, and that had ignited my enthusiasm for working with children in poverty. I spoke at our church and a few other churches in the area and God used that to get sponsors for many children.

Although the public speaking was terrifying to me, the work was incredibly rewarding. It was an amazing feeling to help each child find a sponsor. I was able to travel with a group of Compassion volunteers to the Dominican Republic for training and see their work firsthand. It was so inspiring to see how Compassion truly changes the lives of children living in poverty. The highlight was getting to meet two of our sponsored children and spend the day with them! It was an experience I will never forget.

It truly set me on fire for mission work. I wanted to tell anyone and everyone who would listen not just about what Compassion was doing, but about poverty itself—how it robs children of the ability to dream about a better future. I was easily frustrated by people who seemed indifferent to the harsh reality of poverty. Even though I tried tremendously hard not to look down on people, I did it anyway. I couldn't comprehend knowing—even if it was just head knowledge—about how people in poverty are forced to live and choosing to do nothing about it. How could people stand there with their $5 coffee in hand, shake their heads as if saddened by what they were hearing and then say they couldn't afford to help?

Although I knew it wasn't my place to judge, it ate me up inside.

Even with such a passion for changing the lives of children in poverty, it was still hard for me to ask people to help. I couldn't stand putting people on the spot or asking anyone for help with anything. When I put myself out there and tried to find support for these children, I was really putting my heart on my sleeve. It felt like part of my heart lived with these kids. I imagined what life would look like for the kids we sponsored if they didn't have Compassion in their lives. I imagined how I would feel if Aiden or Noah were living in the same circumstances. It made me sick to think about it and determined to eliminate that way of living for as many children as I could.

Overall, this was a rewarding and peaceful time of life. Our youngest, Noah, took naps each day, and although Aiden didn't actually sleep during naptime, he had quiet time in his room. When I could slow myself down from my endless to-do list, I was able to have quiet time to pray and study. Life seemed so busy, but I didn't realize that I had yet to understand the true meaning of the word.

The more work I did with Compassion, the stronger drive I had to do more tangible work. Something that I could touch and feel in my day-to-day life. Greg and I felt strongly impressed to become foster parents. We went through the whole foster care process, and all that was left was a 12-week class that we needed to take.

Sadly, the class never came available in our area. We asked if we could take it in another county and the social worker said she would try to set it up for us ... but she never did. After many months of asking and trying, we felt pretty discouraged and figured that if fostering was what God truly wanted, then He would have to make it happen.

The foster care process never came to fruition, and we decided that we wanted to have another child. I had a miscarriage between having the boys, so we figured we should get things started earlier rather than later. We still planned to adopt, and I started to think about that a lot, too. That was something that I wanted to do no matter how many kids we had, and I was a little concerned that maybe we would feel like the house was too full after three kids and never move forward with adoption. I did not want that to happen.

However, we were surprised when I became pregnant very quickly this time around. We were super excited!

But it didn't last long. Christmas Eve brought with it intense abdominal pain and the need for monthly supplies. It was not a good Christmas.

As hard as my second miscarriage was, I was still determined to get pregnant again. However, I began thinking about adoption more and more. I'm still not sure why it started to overtake my mind, but, by mid-January, I started to research adoption—"just out of curiosity." I reasoned that if things didn't work out with getting pregnant, then I would have all my ducks in a row for how to start the adoption process.

As time passed, I began to realize that I was hoping I wouldn't get pregnant. This was a pretty shocking realization for someone who had experienced infertility and two miscarriages!

I kept researching and praying and talking to Greg about it. It became all-consuming. One day I decided that I needed to have some serious prayer time with God about the whole situation. That prayer time turned out to be the most incredible encounter with God that I've ever had. I told God what I was thinking and feeling, and asked Him a ton of questions.

And you know what? He answered every single question I asked, over and over and over again. And He would answer in a way that made it perfectly clear that it was not my mind running away with me; it was undeniable that it was Him who was speaking. It was the most amazing, unbelievable time—yet it felt like the most natural thing I've ever experienced. It was life with God the way it was meant to be.

And I had my answer.

That evening, Greg called me on his way home from work. "I don't know how to tell you this, but I had a talk with God today ... and, uh, He wants us to adopt a baby girl from Rwanda ... NOW."

" ... Okay. We'll start the paperwork tonight."

I mean, can I get a hallelujah?! How many men would respond like that?

My husband kinda rocks.

We filed the application with our adoption agency that same night.

A couple weeks later, Greg was in the midst of studying for his boards that physician assistants had to take every six years and the long list of needed adoption paperwork had just been laid out before us in all of its complicated glory.

Then, I got a call.

"Mrs. Maddox, this is the social worker. We have a 4-month-old baby boy who needs placement immediately."

It took a moment for my mind to process this. My brain was in Rwandan adoption mode, and I wasn't catching on that this was the United States calling.

"Wait a second. We never finished the process to become foster parents. There was a 12-week class that we never took."

"I understand that, but you are qualified in an emergency situation, and this *is* an emergency. We have a 4-month-old African American baby boy who needs immediate placement."

"What do you mean by immediate?"

"What time will you be home?"

I arrived home about 90 minutes later, and did my best to explain to a 4 ½-year-old and an almost 2-year-old what was happening. Ten minutes after that, two social workers were at our door, and we had a four-month-old baby.

We were kind of in shock, to say the least.

Our foster son was absolutely precious. He was so happy, and he smiled all the time. It was a tough job juggling three kids that were so young. I was entirely unprepared. It was exhausting—not just physically, but emotionally as well.

After he had been with us for just a couple days, my friend Jade called to see how things were going.

"Pretty well," I said. "But I can tell that I'm holding back emotionally. I'm afraid to give myself to him 100% since I know that this relationship can't last."

"Hmmm ..." replied Jade's sweet voice, "I'm glad God doesn't treat us that way."

Talk about a slap in the face. But it was just the slap that I needed. And Jade is one of those friends who can deliver that slap in love. If someone else said the same thing, you would be offended, hurt and quite possibly be stewing about it for days. Somehow, when Jade reveals a harsh reality, it leaves you pondering and learning from it for years to come.

With one sentence, Jade knocked down all the walls I had built around my heart. After hearing her convicting dose of truth, I committed to giving my heart 100% to that sweet boy.

Years later, at times that I need it most, I can still feel the convicting, beautiful sting of her slap. When dealing with people with whom I'm tempted to think, "They'll never get it," or, "Trying to help them is pointless," I think about how God gives Himself fully, 100%, to every single one of us, regardless of whether or not we ever "get it" or if we choose to believe in Him so our relationship can "last."

It is hard to put into words the enormous stress of this time, both physically and emotionally. Taking care of three small kids while working extra days to help pay for the adoption, Greg studying for boards and trying to make sense of adoption paperwork late every night was simply exhausting.

Additionally, Greg and I could never have a break because a foster child isn't allowed to stay with family or other babysitters. We were beyond drained. On top of it all, here we had a child we fiercely loved—who wasn't ours—yet the child who *is* ours was halfway across the world, and we could do nothing for her.

It was quite the paradox, and it took a toll.

Loving a foster child must be the cruelest form of love there is. It is painful love. Even the happy moments bring so much hurt.

When I found joy in his little firsts and smiles, or when he found joy in me, it was painful. Knowing that the relationship would be broken and that I had no way to explain any of it to him was brutal. It made me angry when people would say things like, "Oh I admire you. I could never do that. I'd get too attached."

I wanted to scream back, "Yeah, because I'm not attached at all. When this kid leaves here, I'll be like, 'See ya! It's been real!'"

Foster parents don't foster because we are somehow immune to getting attached. We foster because it isn't about us and our desire to be comfortable. It's about a kid who needs to be safe and protected and loved. It's a kid who needs to be able to form loving relationships and attachments while in the foster system so that they will know how to do the same once they are out.

Although I wouldn't have actually said those things to someone at the time, and despite the fact that those things are true, they represented my frustrated, exhausted, intolerant attitudes toward people who, in my opinion, couldn't look past themselves.

In fact, when I looked around me, that's mostly what I saw: people who couldn't look past themselves. I was in survival mode; so tired that it made me feel jaded ... and isolated. No one understood me, and I didn't understand anyone else. It's an odd conundrum when you attempt to put yourself aside to care for others, it can make you pull into yourself more.

The agony of the adoption process just added to these feelings all the more.

Something amazing happens when you make the decision to adopt. You go from just dreaming of the possibility to a sudden, shocking realization: I have a child on the other side of the world. I don't know who she is, but God does. She is mine, and I can't take care of her. Only God can. You feel very much pregnant, yet you can't pick out baby clothes because you don't know her age or size. You don't even know what season it will be when you finally bring her home. You can't have checkups to be sure your baby is okay; you can't hear her heartbeat or feel her kick.

Yet, you love her no less.

Some people simply do not—and will not—understand this. They wonder how you can feel such deep pain over a child who remains faceless. Yet the pain is so palpable that you are easily overstimulated by innocuous comments. Comments such as, "It must be so awesome not to have to go through another pregnancy." I've been through both, and I would take the pregnancy any day.

Sometimes you feel angry that no one understands your grief; no one considers you to be expecting. You crave the company of someone who gets your pain, but no one can truly understand unless they are also adopting. You can ask any family that is in the waiting stage: The pain is very real and ever-present, brimming just under the surface of smiles and common courtesies. The heart is always ready to burst, and often does—just not always at times that it is seen by others.

Yet, I fully believe that this pain is a blessing. It is hard, REALLY hard, to see it at the time. But all of this pain is part of what endears you to a child who did not grow in your womb. All of this heartache is what makes you fiercely protective of a child you have not even met. The longing seals the fact that this child, faceless though she may be, is your child. YOUR child. Truly, 100% yours. She may not look like yours, but the motherly instincts and the love in your heart scream otherwise.

It is also a huge lesson in learning to trust God and depending on Him to be your child's comforter. The pain, the longing and the helplessness all seem to throw you headlong into the arms of the only one who can truly be there for her—her Maker.

I lived for updates from our adoption agency, but each one would turn out to be more and more discouraging. Each and every report indicated a longer wait. Just before Thanksgiving, I posted an update on Facebook letting everyone know that nothing would happen until May, at the very earliest.

The Monday after Thanksgiving I checked my email at work, and immediately started screaming. My coworkers all came running to see what was wrong. They found me crying and shaking uncontrollably as I looked at the face of the most beautiful baby girl I had ever seen.

There is always more going on than meets the eye. We think we know so much—we gather all our intel and study to be knowledgeable, but we can never, ever, see the full picture of what God is up to behind the scenes. We just can't. I thought that I truly understood this fact on that day; the day that I first saw my daughter's gorgeous face.

But I still had quite a few lessons looming on my horizon.

⸺⸻⸺

During our time of fostering, I began to notice that I'd get a little dizzy now and then. It was no big deal. I'd just get a little lightheaded or see stars when getting up from tying the boys' shoes or playing with them on the floor. It's one of those things that you think is a little odd, but as a mom, you just don't have time to deal with it. The feelings would come and go, but overall, it was gradually getting worse. It was then that I started to have ringing in my ears and dizziness when I turned my head.

Still, it was mild so it was something that I would not have worried about too much, but we were headed to Rwanda soon. I was concerned about the possibility of an inner ear issue, and since I didn't want anything to happen on the trip or have to worry about running to any doctors once I was back home with our daughter, I decided to see an ENT (Ear, Nose and Throat doctor).

He checked me out and mentioned the possibility of Meniere's disease, which is an inner ear problem that can cause a spinning sensation and ringing in the ears. He set up a test called an ECOG (electrocochleography), which measures electrical potentials generated in the inner ear. I was a little annoyed at the need to return for another test, but I obliged. The testing was all normal, and as the trip approached, my symptoms seemed to lessen.

This was especially surprising considering the absolute grief and exhaustion that we were going through at the time. Just one week before leaving for Africa to get our daughter, we had to say goodbye to our foster son. That was easily one of the worst days of my life. I hate even writing about it because the searing pain comes back afresh. I need more tissues than brain cells as I hash this out on my keyboard!

He was 14 months old at the time. He'd been with us for 10 months, and he called me Mama. He didn't know any better; he was just following what Aiden and Noah did. He didn't know he wasn't a permanent member of our family. We were the only family he knew, and I had no way to explain to him what was happening.

How do you hug and kiss a baby goodbye—in front of your five and two-and-a-half-year-old—knowing it's for good? I remember trying to sear an imprint into my memory of what his little body felt like in my arms as I squeezed him tight before passing him to the social worker. As the tears streamed down my face, I told myself just to let him go, but then I ran after her and grabbed him back as she was walking to her car. I just had to hold him once more.

"That's not going to help, Cristy," she sighed.

"Maybe not," I eked out through my tears, "but he is used to me putting him in his car seat. Not you. I want him to feel safe right now." I hugged him tight, buckled him in his seat, gave him a big smile and a tickle and said, "I love you always, sweet bear." Then I turned and ran into the house sobbing.

Fortunately, my mom was there to take the boys with her and distract them. I don't think I've ever felt such intense pain; I didn't think I would be able to keep breathing. And as much as I hurt, I couldn't bear thinking about what must be going on inside his little head. Was he wondering where I was? When he cried did he expect to see my face leaning over his crib?

I don't know how I would have made it through if we were not going to meet our daughter, Carrington, so soon. The grief was overwhelming, but the joy looking forward was also overwhelming. When I thought about Carrington, my heart was revived, and we did our best to focus on and invest in the boys. They had been through a lot themselves, and we wanted to make them feel as secure as we could before we disappeared to Rwanda for 17 days.

Those 17 days would turn out to be beautiful beyond description. We traveled with eight other incredible families who were also adopting. Talk about a bonding experience! I had found my camaraderie with people who got me; people who knew my passion *and* my pain. And meeting our daughter for the first time ... there is just no way to describe it. But this was my attempt the night after we met.

> Today was THE day. The day that all our hopes over the last year came true. The day that we could set aside what our imaginations have said and embrace the reality before us. The day that we could stop just looking at pictures and reading books about our daughter's place of birth, because now we are walking its streets. The day that we can stop our obsession with studying our daughter's pictures and trying to imagine what she is like in person, because now we know. We know how big she is. We know what her cry sounds like. We know how smooth her skin feels. We know the depth of her eyes. We know the joy that she brings and the depth of the love that God has given us for her. We also know that there is so much more to learn about our beautiful baby, and we can't wait to get started.

Needless to say, I didn't sleep much that night! I couldn't wait to race back to her the next morning. It was a long trip with a lot of time for us to bond one-on-one with Carrington, and we fell head-over-heels in love with her and Rwanda. Rwanda is absolutely stunning, with beautiful, welcoming people to match.

However, it was difficult being so far away from our young boys for such an extended period. Throughout the adoption process, I had been longing for Carrington. When we were gone, I was longing for Aiden and Noah. When we finally arrived back at Richmond International Airport, I collapsed onto the floor and into the arms of my boys with poor Carrington in one arm, staring at these little blond heads that were suddenly bobbing all around her.

The emotion that overwhelmed me was unlike anything else I've ever felt. Such joy and such sweet relief. I hadn't realized the extent of the tension that had built up inside over the previous year until it all flowed out once I had *all* of my babies in my arms.

The joy and relief followed for quite some time. After having a foster son I knew I would lose, the feeling of having all of my kids home, knowing that they were all *mine* and that no one could take them away was indescribable. I had peace inside for the first time in what felt like forever. Constant worry and fear were no longer my companions.

Even though our home was a total circus, our family brought us such joy. After a 12-week adoption leave, I jumped back into my regular routine of work, exercise and caretaking. I was on the go nonstop taking care of the kids, preparing to homeschool Aiden and already starting to plan our next adoption.

Once things settled down just a bit, I wanted to start up my work with Compassion again. We had also come home from Rwanda determined to go back. We truly missed it and knew we wanted to live there—at least for a couple years. With both of our medical backgrounds, I knew we could find a way to serve.

I was happy, strong and confident. God had led so clearly up until now, and although it had not been easy, it had brought me to a place of such joy. There was no reason to think He wouldn't continue to do the same.

I just knew we were right on track to fulfilling the rest of our dreams.

Chapter Two

Someone Else to Somebody

"This is the kind of thing that you always think
will happen to someone else ... but I guess
everyone is someone else to somebody."
— Aiden Maddox, 11 years old

I have seen a lot of painful stories in my years as a physical therapist. My heart breaks for so many patients and families who have suffered so deeply. You can't work in a hospital without being reminded every single shift of the mortality of the life we lead.

Yet somehow, even with the fragility of the human body on display all around me; even with a lump in my throat and tears that threaten to fall as I watch the narratives of others unfold, I never thought it could happen to me. We all say things like, "Life is short. Make the most of it. Enjoy every moment. Don't take anything for granted."

We have a tendency to say so many beautiful, stupid clichés that really don't mean a thing to us. We think we know what we're saying, and we may think it is helpful, but we actually have no clue.

On the other hand, there are plenty of times where we receive well-meaning, encouraging advice, but it won't fully sink in until we're living it out. I think about the time when I was pregnant with Aiden. People kept telling me to enjoy my sleep. "Get plenty of sleep now, because once that baby is here, you won't be able to get much."

"Oh, I will!" I'd respond enthusiastically.

I thought I was enjoying my sleep. I thought I appreciated it. And thinking about being up in the night with my newborn seemed so poetic. The exhausted mother, sacrificing even the basics of life for the undying love she has for her child. (Exhale a contented, dreamy sigh.)

And then he arrived. And that little terror did not sleep. I mean never.

Okay, so that's an exaggeration. He slept if I was driving the car, or bouncing him vigorously, or making shushing sounds in his ear or trying to nurse him. But sleep on his own? Forget about it.

And I thought to myself, *Why didn't anyone tell me how little sleep I would get?! Why didn't they tell me how hard this would be?*

Oh, but they did. I just didn't understand. I repeated what they said with full agreement, but had no idea what that agreement actually meant.

I think the same is true of us when we look at the crises and trials that happen to others. We might *say* that we understand that they could happen to us. We *think* we believe it.

Until it actually happens to us. And we realize that we never truly embraced our own mortality and weakness. We never truly appreciated all our blessings and abilities. We never realized that they are not rights that we are entitled to.

The sad truth is that the only way to know it—to know in your bones how precious and special every single moment and every single tiny ability is—is to have them taken away.

———∞∞∞———

Once Carrington was home, we had a couple of good, intensely busy years of normalcy. Well, as normal as they can be when you are a homeschooling family touched by the loss of a foster child.

Our boys were confused and insecure due to an apparent baby switch out, and our daughter needed to make up for lost time. In addition to this, our two littlest littles were both all about their mama and fought over me nonstop. Noah and Carrington certainly had their struggles over who was Mama's baby.

Noah didn't talk for a long time and was very sensory avoidant, so we spent a lot of time going to speech and occupational therapy. Carrington, on the other hand, was extremely sensory *seeking*—which made the combination of the two of them ... well, I think my mom put it best when she said, "You should have named Noah 'dynamite' and Carrington 'fire.'"

Very soon after returning home from Rwanda, the dizziness had returned and continued off and on. But life was rolling along, and I didn't give it much attention until *it* happened. It was the moment that marked the beginning of a new way of life for our family.

It was an April evening in 2012 during holy hour. You know, that sweet hour of quiet you get just after you get all the kids down before you conk out for the night? I was sitting on the sofa, reading a book on how to help my little Tasmanians' sensory issues. Suddenly, I felt incredibly dizzy out of nowhere. My vision blurred as numbness and tingling started down the right side of my body. My right eyelid felt heavy—as if I couldn't keep my eye open—but it looked perfectly normal.

In retrospect, Greg and I are probably a little too chill about things like this, especially with both of us working in the medical field. If this happened to anyone else, I would have told them to go to the emergency room. (And if it happens to you, go to the emergency room!) However, my strength was good, and apart from the obvious, I was so healthy. I was in great shape; there was no way this was a stroke. Besides—it was late. And we had three small kids in bed asleep. I'll admit, perhaps there was a bit of denial that anything could be wrong. So, we decided to wait, and I would make an appointment with a neurologist the next day.

When I woke up the next morning, my right foot was still numb, the dizziness continued, and my vision was slightly blurred in the periphery. The quickest a neurologist could see me was in a few days, but they wanted me to see an ophthalmologist as soon as possible. When I called for an appointment and told them my story, they asked me to come immediately.

But, of course, everything checked out. My eyes were fine.

When it came time for the neurologist appointment, Greg came with me. Several days had passed, and I was still having symptoms. The neurologist seemed nice at first, but when he heard that I only worked one or two days a week, he asked, "Why don't you want to work?" Um, excuse me? Did he not just hear the part about homeschooling and three kids? Working in the medical field, I knew that wasn't a great sign. He was zeroing in on an imagined laziness signal.

He seemed to be trying to brush us off, saying that all my symptoms could be normal. Fortunately, Greg wasn't having it. He told him what a hard worker I was and insisted that if I said there was a problem, then there *was* a problem. Taking a stand for me, he sternly said, "I know my wife. She doesn't make stuff up!" He pushed for an MRI of my brain to rule out multiple sclerosis, and the doctor agreed. Thankfully, the MRI came back normal.

Next, he said he would do an EMG (Electromyogram) of my right leg. During this test, small needles are inserted through the skin into the muscles to measure their responses to nerve stimulation. The EMG was done in his office, and also came back normal. When he came in to tell me the results, he began asking a few more questions, but I could already tell what he was looking for. He wanted to know what I did each day and what my life was like. I told him it was jam-packed with three young kids, homeschooling and running to various therapies.

Bingo! He had his answer.

"Oh, you are very stressed. What you are having is just anxiety. You need to learn to deal with your stress."

"But I don't feel anxious or stressed."

"That doesn't matter. Sometimes anxiety just presents like this and causes stroke-like symptoms."

I left thinking, *For real? Is that the best answer you can come up with?* I get it that doctors do not have all the answers, and I totally respect them when they are willing to state that fact. However, this situation felt like he was making something up to keep from admitting that he simply didn't know what was going on.

Fortunately, I've been around the medical community long enough to know he was wrong. I knew there was more going on and I wasn't willing to settle for the anxiety card being tossed my way. But it did leave me wondering what happens to patients in my situation who don't know any better. Would they walk away and think, *Wow, I didn't know I was handling stress so badly. How do I learn to deal with stress better?* Or would they trust their intuition and dig deeper?

My symptoms persisted for a few weeks before tapering off, and the numbness eventually went away completely. I still had bouts of dizziness off and on, but it was mild overall, and I was becoming accustomed to it. However, I knew in the back of my mind that we hadn't seen the end of it. With the dizziness persisting, combined with the new recent symptoms, Greg and I both knew there was definitely more going on. But with nothing to pinpoint at the moment, life slipped back into its usual routine.

At the end of July, we went to visit friends where we used to live in Ohio. We typically go every summer, but this year we were not intending to make the trip. However, some other plans fell through, so we planned a fairly spur-of-the-moment visit. I was shocked that it all worked out on such short notice—the trip requires coordinating schedules with a lot of different people.

While we were there, we visited a friend, April, who is a physician assistant and was working in dermatology at the time. A bunch of us were showing her little skin issues that our kids had; you know, being annoying by making her work while hanging out in her backyard. We were about to leave when I remembered that I had a spot on my shoulder that I'd been wondering about but hadn't taken the time to get checked out. I didn't want to bother her with it, especially since we'd already asked her a gazillion questions about our kids, but for some reason, I asked her anyway. She said that it didn't look particularly concerning and questioned why I was worried about it.

"It's just changed. I never noticed it before, but this summer it's such a bright pink that sometimes when I wear a sleeveless shirt, I put concealer on it."

"Well, if you think it's changed that much then why don't you just stop by my office while you are here and I'll biopsy it for you?"

Honestly, my only thought was, *Sweet! No co-pay!* Plus, I had childcare readily available with Greg and friends there, and her office was super close to where we were staying. There would be no driving an hour to get to the doctor like I have to do when I'm home. Convenience was really the only thing on my mind. I greatly appreciated her generosity and took her up on it.

When I left her office, I didn't think about it again. That is, until when I was back home in Virginia a week later, and she called me with the results.

"Cristy, first of all, I just want to tell you that you are going to live a long and happy life."

Uh oh. That's not a good start to a conversation. I didn't know my longevity was ever in question.

"The biopsy came back, and it is melanoma. It looks like we caught it early though. You are going to need to find a dermatologist to take this out for you. You will have a three-inch scar on your shoulder, and you'll have to see the dermatologist every three months, but I genuinely believe that we've caught this in time."

Someone Else to Somebody

I couldn't believe it. Not like "freaking out" couldn't believe it, but, "Oh my word, look what I just narrowly avoided! God is so good!" not believing it. I honestly could not get over it. We had not planned that trip, and it came together on short notice. I showed the spot to April on a whim, and she was kind enough to offer to biopsy it when it looked nothing like melanoma! For the record, melanoma is black, not pink.

Yeah, I had been planning to get an appointment with a dermatologist eventually, but I'd done nothing about it, and it takes months to get in with one. By the time I decided to do anything, it would have been too late.

And since I'd done nothing, now I had melanoma, but no dermatologist. April faxed my report to Greg, who was working in primary care at the VA hospital. Greg took it straight to the chief of dermatology at the VA. He looked at the report, picked up the phone and called his buddy, who is a dermatology surgeon in private practice. He explained the situation. Then he handed the phone to Greg, and the guy told him, "I'll do your wife's surgery tomorrow."

Oh, my word. God is good. Still not believing it.

I can't tell you how rare it is to arrive at a doctor's office on surgery day as a new patient. The office staff couldn't figure out what was happening! Where was my chart? How did I get on his surgery schedule if I'd never seen him before?

Despite the confusion, everything went well with the excision. The only problem was they didn't let me see what they were doing. With melanoma, they have to take the tissue all the way down to the muscle—it would have been pretty cool to get a look at my own deltoid.

The report came back showing that the cells on the sides were in the process of changing into melanoma, so a few weeks later we had to do the excision again to take out more tissue. Another chance to see my deltoid; they still didn't let me look. But that was it. Just two excisions and a lifting restriction while it healed. That is a terribly small inconvenience to get rid of cancer!

Honestly, I was mostly concerned that having a cancer diagnosis on my record would hinder us from getting approved to adopt again. I didn't know if it would be a major issue, but I didn't want *anything* to get in our way.

By December of that year, my arm was pretty well healed. We were rolling along in our usual busy holiday routines when I noticed the dizziness beginning to worsen. For the most part, I tried to ignore it, but then I started to have pressure and ringing in my ears along with noise sensitivity. And can I just add, this was *not* funny. I'm the mother of three small kids. The noise *never* stops! I then began to notice that the dizziness would get worse when I saw a lot of movement.

Umm, did I mention the three small children?

One evening I went to Sam's Club with the kids. Greg was on his way from work and would be ready to meet us for dinner about the time we finished with our shopping. We'd only been in the store a minute or two when I noticed everything getting louder and brighter. Carrington was sitting in the shopping cart, and with every single little move she made, I became increasingly dizzier. (And she *never* stops moving!) I was trying to get her to be still while also trying to keep track of the boys, but turning my head to look for them made things worse.

Eventually, I realized that I was getting into real trouble. I was starting to lose my balance to my right side, and I was getting nauseated. We were near the restrooms, and I managed to find a spot where I could lean against the wall. I ordered the boys to stay put and prayed they would. Aiden probably would have tried to help with Carrington if he had a clue what was happening, but he didn't understand. I thought if I rested for a minute that I'd be able to continue—or at the very least, get us out of the store.

But it didn't get better ... it got worse. I could barely stand. I tried to text Greg, but was having trouble figuring out how to send him a message. I finally got something out like, "help bathroom."

It took him a while to get there from work and find us. In the meantime, he was texting me questions to which I couldn't respond. When he did get there, he read the situation quickly. He helped me lean on the cart, started barking orders to the kids and guided us out the door.

Once outside, I started to feel better, but I still wasn't right. My balance and depth perception were very off. I made it safely to my vehicle, but I wasn't able to drive. Needless to say, we weren't too sure what to do. We were twenty-five minutes from home with two cars. We decided that Greg would take the kids to eat at Taco Bell while I rested in the car. I laid my seat back and put my feet up on the dashboard. After about 45 minutes or so, I felt well enough to drive. I drove slowly and cautiously and made it home safely.

For the next several days, the dizziness became worse, and my balance continued to be a problem. At times, my hands would shake, and I felt very uncoordinated. I found myself having a hard time finding the right words to articulate what I was trying to say. I didn't drive for several days because I just didn't feel safe enough to do so, especially with the kids in tow.

As my symptoms worsened—the pressure and ringing in my ears, along with dizziness and imbalance—I decided to return to the ENT. He repeated the ECOG testing, which showed a slight increase in pressure in my right ear, but nothing of real significance. It definitely wasn't diagnostic for Meniere's disease, but something was going on. I seemed to be getting increasingly fatigued, and there were new and worsening symptoms.

I loved my new dermatologist, Dr. Reese, and at my follow-ups for melanoma, she would ask questions about dizziness, headaches and appetite issues. I had a lot of things going on, but since there were no skin changes, it clearly wasn't a recurrence of melanoma. However, she was interested in these symptoms and strongly recommended that I see a neurologist.

At this point, I was over it. I'd gone from almost never seeing a doctor to seeing multiple specialists, going through various tests and having two minor surgeries. Besides, the first neurologist I saw certainly didn't help me any. But she insisted that she knew a very capable one with good bedside manner. I told her that I thought using the words neurologist and good bedside manner in the same sentence was akin to an oxymoron, but I trusted her. And I'm so glad I did!

The neurologist, Dr. Ham, is awesome. Seeing her is like sitting down with a girlfriend—well, a girlfriend who gives you homework. She had me write up a report on myself and everything that had happened, including all my symptoms, every doctor I had seen and every test I had done. Dr. Ham cared enough to ask the probing questions to be sure she understood the full story and told me that she was basically my healthcare detective now. She was the one who would look at the big picture and try to investigate and sort this thing out. I am truly blessed to have had her on my side and believing in me so early on.

She had several things that she wanted to investigate right off the bat. First, she ordered a CTA (an imaging scan of the blood vessels) of my head and neck. Second, she referred me to an ear specialist—someone who only does ears and is more specialized than an ENT. Third, she wanted me to have a sleep study. I really gagged at that third one. A sleep study! Honestly, I thought that was a little over the top, but I was so happy to have someone who sincerely wanted to get to the bottom of what was going on that I would have washed in the Jordan seven times if she'd asked me to.

The CTA ended up coming back normal. The ear specialist also did several tests and came to the conclusion that I was having vestibular migraines. These are migraines that affect the ears, vision and balance without necessarily causing head pain. Finally, I thought we had a simple answer. He put me on medication, but I only stayed on it for six weeks because it caused weakness and increased appetite with no improvement in my symptoms. I would wake up in the middle of the night dying to eat!

I reluctantly went ahead with the sleep study and was shocked to find that I have sleep apnea. There had been no signs of it. I don't snore, and I can't fall asleep unless I have my fan on and all my pillows tucked into place just so. What especially surprised me was how low my oxygen levels were dropping during the night; this was both depressing and hope inducing. *How am I supposed to get used to a stupid CPAP? Will it scare the kids?* But I was also thinking, *Maybe this is it. Maybe this is why I've been feeling so bad. This could sincerely change things.*

The sleep doctor also did allergy testing, and apparently, I am allergic to everything. *Okay, then why am I not dead?* That just sounded stupid to me. How can you be allergic to everything and not even know it, especially when you've never had allergies before? Nonetheless, I started allergy medicine and did the hard work of getting used to the CPAP (a machine used at night to apply air pressure to prevent your airway from collapsing). I was starting to get desperate. I was willing to try just about anything to be able to get some normalcy back into my life.

The CPAP did make a big difference in the number of headaches and dizziness I had, and I felt a lot less tired. I was doing better! I wasn't 100%, but it was a definite improvement. Things were looking up ... at least for a little while.

That seemed to be that pattern of how things would go. I'd seem better for a month or two, and then things would come back with new and worsening symptoms. It made us concerned about where this unidentified thing was headed. I had so many tests and saw so many doctors. It was hard to keep track of it all.

In May of 2013, I was doing fairly well. Due to having sleep apnea, I needed to see a cardiologist, so I set up an appointment with one of my favorite doctors I worked with, Dr. Agyeman. During the appointment, he noticed an irregular heartbeat. He had me wear a 30-day event monitor to see how my heart was doing. One day at work, he pulled me aside to let me know that some of the results concerned him. I returned to my business of seeing my own patients, thinking, *Now I've got heart problems! Are you kidding me?!*

In order to address his concern, Dr. Agyeman ordered a stress test for me. But everything with the test looked normal. When the nurse said that they had gotten enough information, he said, "No, let's see how long she can go. It's not often that we get a patient who can run like this." Apparently, my heart was in great shape. Such good shape, in fact, that the doctor wanted me to keep running even when the test was done because he so rarely got to see a healthy heart in action!

When the test was finished, I asked, "So if everything looks great, do you have *any* ideas as to why I'm getting dizzy with position changes?"

"When you go home, look up POTS. That stands for Postural Orthostatic Tachycardia Syndrome. See if you think that sounds at all like you, and let me know when you see me at work. It would actually be great if it's just POTS; that condition is pretty easy to treat."

I had never heard of POTS before. When I asked Greg about it, he had never heard of it either.

When I looked it up, I learned that POTS can have several different mechanisms, but commonly POTS patients don't get enough blood flow to their brains when they stand up because their blood vessels don't work properly to counteract gravity. Their heart rate increases as they change positions, resulting in symptoms like dizziness, near-fainting, shakiness and balance issues.

POTS is one potential result of dysautonomia, which is a malfunction of the autonomic nervous system (ANS). The

ANS controls all your organs, and basically everything you don't think about doing. Think blood pressure, heart rate, digestion, hormones; the list could go on and on. The listed symptoms sounded all too familiar, so it certainly seemed like POTS could be a possibility.

Except for one thing: the fast heart rate (tachycardia). I didn't struggle with tachycardia, and that seemed to be a key factor for POTS. I was in great cardiovascular shape—the stress test had just proved that!

When I told Dr. Agyeman my thoughts, he said, "Well, there is a simple test we can do to find out. Why don't we set you up for a tilt table test?"

"Okay, why not?"

It's funny to think about how before I had these issues, I would have thought one single test was such a pain! I didn't have any time for things like that, and the expense alone would have been so irritating to me. Now, it was definitely a pain—and the expense was becoming more and more of a problem—but my perspective had changed entirely. This was my life. This was my families' lives. It was my ability to continue doing my job; it was my livelihood.

Besides, I was starting to have more trouble again. The dizziness was increasing, and this time I had fatigue that felt debilitating. I was having weakness in my right leg at times, which was new and concerning, and my balance just wasn't right. I couldn't go into a big store without significant problems, which made me afraid to shop with the kids. I knew I couldn't keep myself safe, much less them. We would get stuck in town because the large stores combined with all of the movements that the kids would make in the shopping carts would make me so dizzy that

I couldn't drive. I'd try to rest in the car until I could drive, but it would take a long time with three littles rocking the van in their car seats.

Later, one of my doctors referred to this as "Walmart Phenomenon." In fact, before I even told him what was happening, he asked if I had all of these symptoms in large stores. He stated that it is a vestibular or inner ear migraine triggered by all the overwhelming sensory input that is typical of warehouse type stores; tall ceilings, bright lights, people moving in all directions, noise, color, smells and wiggling children in shopping carts.

Um, yeah. I could be the poster child for "Walmart Phenomenon." Just don't put me on People of Walmart.

One night in Home Depot, my right leg was literally dragging. I couldn't get my toes to clear the floor. It looked like I was having a stroke. I was also having episodes where my heart rate dropped in the low 50s with activity, which made me feel like I could barely stand up.

With my heart rate being too low, I felt pretty convinced that I didn't have POTS. I decided to put off the tilt table test because I needed to have a small surgery. In addition to the other issues, I'd been having frequent abdominal pain this whole time. Since my mother had a history of endometriosis (a condition in which the lining of the uterus grows on other pelvic organs), we suspected I might as well. When I was in college, she had one of the worst cases of endometriosis that her doctors had ever seen. Her surgery was quite extensive.

My surgery was minor. It was mainly for diagnostic purposes so we could determine how to treat the problem—I probably would have put it off until the pain was much more severe had it not been for my family history. The surgery went well; it confirmed that I had endometriosis, but it took me a long time to wake up from the anesthesia. I could hear the nurses talking and saying, "Her heart rate is in the 30s again." I'd think, *Well that's not good*, and conk back out. It happened several times, and I remember they kept giving me medication to bring it back up. I was awake but couldn't open my eyes.

It left me wondering if it was a reaction to the anesthesia or if there was something legitimately going on with my heart.

Soon after this, I started having numbness in my right hand and difficulty grasping a pen. My hand would start cramping, and it fatigued incredibly fast with any activity. It would start to tremor, and I'd drop items I had been holding. Once I was moving a metal folding chair across the room and nearly smashed Greg's acoustic guitar when I dropped it. The noise was loud, and Greg and I locked eyes with each other, both thinking, *What is happening?*

We were both becoming concerned about the same thing: Lou Gehrig's disease. Even saying it out loud was scary. I thought, *Anything but that, God. I'll take any other diagnosis but that!* Sometimes we have just enough medical knowledge to cause us to be too relaxed about medical issues, and sometimes we have just enough knowledge to freak ourselves out.

Just three days after surgery, we went on our annual summer trip. We go for a week of summer camp together as a family, and our friends from Ohio join us. It is held in the mountains of Virginia, and everywhere you go there are tons of hills to walk up and down. When we went the year before in 2012, I had hiked all over with three-and-a-half-year-old Carrington on my back and I'd hardly gotten out of breath.

By 2013, there was a drastic difference; I was so embarrassed by how poor my balance was. I was the only person who was thrilled that it rained most of the week because I could use our umbrella as a cane on those hills and no one realized its true purpose. My right leg was just too weak and numb to be stable enough in that setting. When we went hiking, I had to use an actual cane, which absolutely mortified me. I was embarrassed for Greg to see me with it, much less all these families that we'd see at camp each year.

In mid-July, I finally got around to following through with the tilt table test. They strapped me to a table, and I rested there for several minutes while my vital signs were monitored. Then they tilted the table upright and continued to monitor my heart rate and blood pressure for 20 minutes. I didn't feel very good, but was okay throughout the whole test, and my vitals looked fine. I was thinking, *Well this was a waste of time.*

Dr. Agyeman told me that everything was normal, and that they were just going to lay me back down and monitor my vitals for a few more minutes before we'd be finished. As they laid the table down, I suddenly became incredibly dizzy. Before I could even say anything, Dr. Agyeman was asking, "What's going on Crystal? What are you feeling?" He was leaning over me and looking at the monitors; I could tell he was legitimately concerned.

"I'm really dizzy, and my feet are numb, but my heels are burning."

It wasn't the first time I had felt that way. In fact, it wasn't terribly unusual for me to feel that way when I changed positions.

Oddly enough, it was sometimes more severe when I laid down after being on my feet a while.

"Your blood pressure dropped from the 120s to 90 immediately, and your heart rate went from the 90s to 50." I could tell he was flustered. "You just did the *exact opposite* of what I was expecting you to do during this test!"

What *I* thought was strange was that my heart rate had been in the 90s while standing. That was quite high for me. "What does that mean?"

"I don't know! It means ... it means you're an alien ... and that I am not smart enough to figure you out. I need to refer you on to that highly respected electrophysiologist in Richmond that I mentioned to you before."

I gotta say, I have mad respect for doctors who admit when they don't know what's going on. I mean, Dr. Agyeman could have told me I was having anxiety! I much preferred being called an alien.

———

Throughout the rest of the summer, I began to notice that the weakness in my right side would get worse anytime I was out in the heat. On a trip to visit friends in Ohio and my sister in Indiana, I was limping most of the time. If I was out in the heat, the limp got even worse. I made the mistake of getting in a hot tub once, and I didn't think I would even be able to walk afterward. This made us more concerned about multiple sclerosis. My first MRI was normal, but we'd done more research and wondered if it had just been too early for it to show. I was thankful that Dr.

Ham had set me up with a neuro-ophthalmologist soon after we returned home.

But then another strange symptom appeared. One morning while staying at a friend's house in Ohio, I got up and walked up a half flight of stairs and was suddenly completely out of breath, feeling like my heart was racing. I took my heart rate, and it was in the 120s. From half a flight of steps?!

Conveniently, the friend we were staying with is a physician assistant who works in cardiology. (Do I have awesome hook-ups with my friends, or what?) So, we took off for his office, and he did an electrocardiogram. By then my heart rate had returned to normal, and everything looked fine. From that point forward, these episodes started to happen more and more frequently.

I was super anxious for the appointment with the neuro-ophthalmologist. It had taken a long time to get the appointment, and Dr. Ham seemed to think that he would have some answers. Greg came with me because he was getting quite concerned with all the weakness and limping. (Plus, I'd almost smashed his guitar because of my hand!) The doctor was severely lacking in bedside manner, but I figured I could overlook that if he knew his stuff. He wasn't terribly concerned about multiple sclerosis since the first MRI was normal, but he did want to repeat the MRI. He wanted to rule out strokes, cerebral vasculitis and myotonic dystrophy.

Even for a couple of medical professionals, there were a lot of big possibilities to process on the spot. However, he thought the most likely scenario was a complex migraine. He said that there are many forms of migraine, even hemiplegic ones that cause stroke-like symptoms. It made sense, considering it often happened in situations that would typically trigger migraines in people. He was starting me on aspirin just in case strokes were an issue, as well as a migraine medication.

It should have been a bit of a relief having a fairly mild diagnosis on the table and a plan to rule out the bigger stuff. But I left his office in tears because he was so condescending and rude. At one point, he was testing sensation in my face with a tuning fork. After hitting the tuning fork to make it vibrate, he tested the left side of my forehead, but then he turned and talked to his medical student for a while before placing it on the right side. He then asked if it felt the same or less than the other side. I said, "Less, but ..." I was going to say that it was no longer vibrating, but he had already turned to the student and was telling him that basically some of this was in my head because the skull will transfer the vibration sense even if there were lack of sensation.

Excuse me?! I was so shocked and angry that he would say that in front of me that I was at a loss for words. Even if I *could* get any words out, he wasn't giving me a chance to talk anymore. It seemed that since he thought it was in my head, he no longer wanted to hear anything that Greg or I had to say. If we tried to jump in, he cut us off. I was trying very hard not to cry in front of him. It wasn't in my head. It was an incorrectly administered test! It was doctor malfunction! And he didn't even give his patient a chance to explain. I never wanted to see him again. Ever.

Once we got in the car, I could not stop crying. I sobbed and sobbed. Greg couldn't figure out why I was taking it so hard. He thought that I was scared of the big diagnoses we were trying to rule out with the tests that were ordered. That wasn't it at all. I knew those bigger issues were probably unlikely. But I also knew how collaboration happened within a hospital system, and I could only imagine what that doctor was going to write in my chart. Making it up? Needs to see Psych? I was now established with several good doctors within his network, and I knew that whatever he wrote would follow me wherever I went. What if Dr. Ham saw the results of that test and no longer believed in me? I was afraid that I'd no longer have anyone on my side. Doctors have no idea the power they have to absolutely crush their patients.

Fortunately, all of the testing came back normal—even an expensive test for myotonic dystrophy. I was starting to think that maybe migraines were all that was going on, but I didn't understand why I was so exhausted and weak all the time. Weren't migraines supposed to go away at some point?

Then I began having burning and an electrical type pain in my feet, and my heart rate started becoming faster with less and less activity. It could be in the 140s with changing the laundry, and it made the simplest things so hard to do. Sometimes just standing to fix dinner seemed like the most monumental task in the world. On the other hand, there were times when my heart rate was in the 40s, leaving me lightheaded and feeling as if I'd pass out. It was all so unpredictable.

When I discussed the heart rate issues and burning in my feet with Dr. Ham, she said that she was starting to think that this wasn't a neurological issue. I started to panic, thinking that she was giving up on me and wanted me off her caseload. Had she read the rude, know-it-all doctor's incorrectly administered test? If it's not neurological, then there is no need for a neurologist, right? She thought it could be some form of dysautonomia. I had heard the term. I knew I'd seen it somewhere as I was researching what was wrong with me, but at that point, I couldn't remember where or what it was. She wanted me to see Dr. Sica. He is a nephrologist (kidney doctor). I didn't have a clue as to why I would need one of those, but she said that he is the expert on dysautonomia.

"Okay. Whatever you think is best."

What choice did I have? I was skeptical. I did *not* like that last specialist she sent me to, and although he had ruled out some diagnoses, we still didn't know what was going on for sure. It sounds ridiculous, but I felt a bit like I was being abandoned. Being sick makes you feel so completely vulnerable, and Dr. Ham was my lifeline.

"I also want to do a skin test on your right leg for small fiber neuropathy. If you do in fact have dysautonomia, you may have some damage to your nerves. That would explain the burning in your feet, and partially explain why your right leg feels so weak. Small fiber neuropathy skews your sensation, and therefore your perception of what is going on in that area. It can make the weakness much more pronounced or exaggerated."

"So where do I get that test done?"

"Right here. I'll do it. I'll have to numb a couple spots on your leg to take a sample of tissue, and it will take it a little while to heal. The results won't come back for a couple of weeks, but it's done right here."

She wasn't dropping me!

"So, I'll still be seeing you?"

"Yes, I'm still managing your case right now. We will see what Dr. Sica has to say, but I'm still on board as long as you need me."

After the last doctor she had sent me to, I was very nervous about seeing Dr. Sica. When I met him, it took about two seconds for all of that worry to dissipate. Dr. Sica is like a sweet old teddy bear, and he greets you with twinkling eyes and a big hug. He took orthostatics, which is heart rate and blood pressure in lying, sitting and standing positions, and took a thorough history.

He looked at the results of my tilt table test and said, "Your heart rate and blood pressure do not follow any pattern known to humankind."

"Well, that makes sense, because Dr. Agyeman called me an alien."

He asked me a lot of questions that made me wonder if he had cameras in my house watching me.

"Do you have trouble when you first stand up in the morning? Do you get dizzy and weak when you take a shower? Do you feel worse when you go outside in the heat? Do you have a hard time standing in place, like in line at the grocery store? Does your heart rate skyrocket like you're doing a cardio workout with simple things like fixing dinner?"

How did he know that all of these things were SO hard for me? It had gotten to the point where my heart rate would sometimes go as high as the 160s when I stood up in the morning. I was having a hard time showering, and sometimes washed my hair over the side of the tub and then took a bath instead of standing in the shower. All of my symptoms were worse in the heat, and standing in place was the cruelest form of torture I could imagine. The only thing that seemed to surprise him was that I was also having bouts of low heart rate as well.

Then he said it. "It certainly sounds like you have some form of dysautonomia. Your tilt table test wasn't diagnostic for POTS, although it does show autonomic dysfunction. But POTS can easily be missed with one test. POTS would not explain your low heart rate, but you could have some conduction abnormalities and POTS will make any underlying condition worse. Sometimes the diagnosis is made based on overall symptoms and patterns of heart rate rather than on an individual test. There are some things that we can try to see how you respond, and this will help to either make the diagnosis or rule it out."

I was trying to take it all in, and a million questions were running through my mind. I wished Greg were there to help me ask the right ones. Plus, I just didn't think he was going to believe this. Could we finally be narrowing in on a real diagnosis; one that wasn't super scary and made sense of everything? Hadn't Dr. Agyeman said that POTS was easy to treat?

This seemed just too good to be true.

However, I was a bit surprised at what Dr. Sica wanted to try. Most of my life, I had avoided medication as much as possible, and tried to use natural remedies whenever I could. Now, I'd do anything that gave me hope of functioning normally again. I was fully expecting for him to start talking about medications, so when he told me that he wanted me to do home infusions of saline twice a week, I wasn't sure what to think. Although I wanted to know the purpose first, I mostly just needed to know the logistics. Once I had those questions satisfied, all I wanted to know was how fast I could start and how soon we would know if this was providing any answers!

Dr. Sica set up for a home health nurse to come to my home and place an IV so I could start the infusions. All the supplies were delivered ahead of time, including the IV pump with a convenient backpack so I could go about my business of taking care of kids and homeschooling while running my infusions. The nurse taught me how to operate the pump and start and stop my IV so I could do it all myself on my own timetable. I just needed her to place the IV once a week with three kids circling her while she did it. I'd keep it in for a few days until I infused my second bag of saline, then I'd remove the IV.

So, about half of my days I had an IV in my arm that I was trying to keep dry and hidden. Most of the nurses were good about putting it in my forearm so that bending my elbow or wrist did not affect it, but occasionally they couldn't find a vein, and I'd end up with one in my wrist or hand. That was tricky to cover and explain to other people in public. I was certain I was going to end up on People of Walmart. (Yeah, I don't know what's up with my fear of winding up on People of Walmart. Maybe if you followed my kids and me around the store for a few minutes you'd understand.)

Because with many cases of POTS your blood vessels do not constrict when you stand to prevent your blood from following gravity, the infusions should help by increasing the volume your heart has available to pump, making it easier to get the blood up to your heart and brain. Even though this treatment was just a simple bag of IV saline, it did help a lot. The weakness, dizziness and fatigue lessened for about 48 hours after an infusion.

The problem with the IVs—besides the fact that they only provide temporary relief—is that they are a huge pain to keep up with for long. Just dealing with getting deliveries and nursing out to your house with three kids can be an ordeal in itself! Not to mention the fact that you are living with an IV in your arm (and trying to not get it wet), giving yourself the infusions, and ridiculous copays. Yet, even with the hassle, I wanted to continue because they made me feel *so* much better.

Because the infusions made such a big difference, I stopped them several days before a couple of tests that were coming up. I was set up for testing with the highly respected electrophysiologist (EP doctor) that Dr. Agyeman sent me to after the wacky tilt table test. I did not want the extra fluid to make things appear far better than they were. As it turns out, Dr. Sica works with and knows this EP doctor quite well, and he was delighted that I was going to repeat a tilt table and stress test with him.

By now it was October, four months after my first stress test—which had shown that my heart was in great shape. I hadn't had any good days in a long time, but the morning of the stress and tilt table test I woke up with my heart rate at only 100. *Great*, I thought, *Of all the days to have a good day. I hope the doctor sees what he needs to see.* The EP doctor wasn't there for the stress test portion, but one of his nurse practitioners was present. I hit my target heart rate for my age during the warmup, so it didn't take long before they were ready to stop the test. Honestly, I was ready to stop, too. Although I could push through the fast heart rate for a while, my right leg was starting to give out.

Next, I was to have the tilt table test, but there was a long wait in between tests, so my heart rate had plenty of time to calm down. The EP doctor was there for part of the test, but he seemed highly irritated. He looked at my vitals a few times while I was in a standing position. He commented more than once that my heart rate was only 95. Meanwhile, I was feeling lightheaded and thankful that I was strapped to the table because my right leg felt so weak. Nevertheless, he wasn't impressed.

A normal heart rate is between 60 and 100, so I wasn't out of a normal range. However, *my* normal just a couple months prior to this was in the 60s when standing. It had gone from 70 up to 110 when they first stood me up, but that was before the doctor graced me with his presence, and nothing dramatic happened this time when they laid me back down.

Everything was normal according to the test standards, but everything did not seem normal with the doctor. I suppose since he was so highly respected he was used to getting more exciting cases than I had turned out to be that particular day.

Gruffly, he said, "Mrs. Maddox, everything is completely normal with all of the tests we have run today." Then he motioned me toward the door.

I was completely flustered and am sure I was red in the face. "How can they be normal when I reached my heart rate max so fast?"

"They *are* normal. They just show a deconditioned heart. You need to exercise more."

He should have taken my heart rate at that moment, because I'm sure it was at a much more exciting rate after that comment.

"But that was my biggest complaint when I came to you in the first place!" My voice was beginning to crack. "I exercise five days a week. I always have, and nothing has changed, except that now my heart is *acting* like it is deconditioned when it has absolutely no reason to be!"

"I don't know what to tell you, Mrs. Maddox. You just need to exercise more." And with that, he motioned me to the door again.

I'm sure my face looked like a tomato at that point, but what else could I say? I couldn't believe this guy. Mr. highly respected, well-known and sought-after physician, and that is the best you can do? I'm a homeschooling mother of three who also works part-time, and exercising five days a week isn't enough?

I found myself in the same position I had been in before—afraid that Dr. Sica would not believe in me anymore after reading this doctor's notes. I was scheduled to return to Dr. Sica after he received the results of the tests, so I knew he was going to be looking at them.

Plus, I needed to see Dr. Sica because my veins were beginning to give out. It was becoming harder and harder for the nurses to find a spot to put the IV. Dr. Sica had said that if we were going to continue infusions long term, then we were going to have to consider putting a port-a-cath in my chest; the same device that people use for cancer treatments.

As I was driving to the appointment, I felt very concerned. I wasn't sure what we were going to do. I did not want a port-a-cath, yet my veins couldn't hold up to the IVs any longer. I was praying and asking God for guidance, thinking, *What an odd situation to be in*. I've been to other countries where the need for clean water is a daily struggle, but here I was, in America, with all the clean water I could ever want, and I was unable to provide for my *own* hydration needs. I turned on the radio—which I never do because I can't stand the commercials—and immediately stumbled upon a Christian station. They were reading a scripture:

"The Lord will guide you continually, giving you water when you are dry and restoring your strength. You will be like a well-watered garden, like an ever-flowing spring."

– Isaiah 58:11, NLT

Giving you water when you are dry ... God certainly has some good timing.

Sure enough, when I discussed my concerns with Dr. Sica, he had a plan to delay the need for a port-a-cath. We would make some medication changes and tweak some dosages to help me retain more fluid. As he started looking over the results of both tilt table and stress tests and comparing the two, I began to feel nervous. What would he think of what the other doctor wrote?

"Was the EP doctor banging his head against the wall during your test?" he asked.

I was confused. "No. He mostly seemed irritated and wanted to get it over with. Why?"

"Well, I think I told you before, but your heart rate and blood pressure don't follow any known patterns."

"He didn't seem to think that anything was wrong at all. He told me I was just deconditioned and needed to exercise more ... that doesn't make any sense to me, Dr. Sica. There was such a change from my first stress test to the next, and I haven't changed my exercise routine at all, even though it is incredibly tough for me."

"Crystal, your case is not usual because dysautonomia has no usual. Most doctors are thrown off by it because it doesn't fit inside neat parameters, but there are no parameters with dysautonomia.

POTS and dysautonomia are the great masqueraders. They will mimic a thousand other things. If we try to chase down every symptom, we will send you to a hundred doctors and put you through a hundred tests. That is why it's so hard for people to find a correct diagnosis. So, let's get your POTS symptoms under control and then see what symptoms we have left. Those are the symptoms that we will chase. But since we know what you have, now we are going to work toward finding the right combination of treatment to manage your symptoms."

"So ... we do officially know what I have? What are you saying that I have exactly?"

He seemed surprised that I didn't know already. I did, of course, but needed to hear it from his mouth.

"You have dysautonomia and POTS."

CHAPTER THREE

I'm Supposed to be at the Beach

"And we know that God causes all things to work together for good to those who love God, to those who are called according to His purpose."
— Romans 8:28, NASB

Is it strange to want to jump for joy when you're told you have some weird diagnosis?

Yeah, I would have thought that it was too. However, my symptoms began in 2009, and it was now October of 2013. After four years of progressing symptoms causing us to wonder what was going on; going from doctor to doctor and having test after test with no answers, and being told things like "you just have anxiety," it was an unbelievable relief to have a diagnosis. It felt like something to celebrate.

Truth be told, I was one of the lucky ones. In fact, a survey conducted by Dysautonomia International the same year I was diagnosed showed that the average length of time from onset of symptoms to a diagnosis for POTS patients is five years and 11 months.[1] Most patients, like me, go to multiple specialists

---

[1] Dysautonomia International (December 2013). Diagnostic Delay in POTS. Retrieved from http://www.dysautonomiainternational.org/page.php?ID=184

before finding a doctor who knows what POTS is and recognizes the symptoms.

Even though Dr. Agyeman didn't realize at the time how complex POTS is, he did know what it was and made a good assessment early on. Thankfully, there has been a lot of research in recent years. Dr. Agyeman actually stated recently, "It's extremely complex. The more we learn, the more we realize how much we don't know."

Although we still have a long way to go, knowledge is increasing in the medical community, and that makes my heart smile. I don't want other people to doubt themselves the way I did. My problems had gone on so long without a definitive diagnosis that at times I started to wonder if I was losing my mind.

I'd think things like, *Well, I know I had symptoms initially, but maybe now I just think they are still there when they're gone. Could my mind be producing symptoms just because I think something is wrong?* When I wasn't so physically fatigued, I knew this wasn't true, especially because I could see the stark contrast between what I felt in my rested moments and how I felt most of my exhausted, symptom-filled hours. Even still, not feeling like yourself physically does play tricks on your mind.

At other moments, I wondered if everyone else were losing their minds. It became so normal for me to feel bad that I forgot what it was like to feel good. If I was standing around talking with a group of people, typically I'd be feeling absolutely miserable inside. I'd look around and think, *Why do people keep talking? Don't they realize that everyone is exhausted from all this standing by now?! Why doesn't anyone suggest we find somewhere to sit?* I found myself unable to relate to the behaviors and actions of my peers. Being sick had robbed my mind of an understanding of normalcy.

With a diagnosis came relief, largely because it validated that I wasn't crazy; that there was a physical reason behind all the symptoms I was feeling. However, the greatest relief came from knowing that I now had treatment options. You can't treat something if you don't know what it is or where it originated. So, I was elated to have a diagnosis.

Dr. Sica had said that there were many different medications to try, and there were also things I could do to help my symptoms on my own. First of all, I needed to drink a ton of water—all day long, all the time. Well, I wasn't too hopeful that this would help, because I already did this. Next, I needed to eat a lot of salt—and I mean a lot. He recommended that I consume ten grams (or 10,000 milligrams) of sodium a day.

To put that in perspective, the American Heart Association recommends no more than 2,300 milligrams a day, and an ideal limit of 1,500 milligrams. For most people, too much sodium can contribute to heart disease. But with POTS, the more sodium you eat, the more fluids you retain, and having more fluids means that more blood makes it to your heart and brain. I could also use waist-high compression stockings. Although not the most fashionable—and way too hot to wear in the summer—they do provide a lot of relief during the colder months. They help keep much of my blood from dropping to my legs, and as a result, my heart rate is lower.

My workouts were something else that needed to change, but I couldn't accept it. I had always done very intense workouts five or more days a week. It was my stress relief, and the only way I could seem to somewhat keep my weight down. Plus, with POTS it is incredibly important to have very strong leg muscles because they help to compensate for the lack of tone in the blood vessels and assist with pumping the blood.

However, now when I did an intense cardio workout, my heart rate was in the 190s all throughout. Not only was it completely miserable for every single second of the workout, but I couldn't recover afterward. My heart rate would stay up—sometimes in the 120s or more for a couple of hours afterward, even if I sat to rest. Then I would have no energy left for the rest of the day.

I knew I needed to alter my routine, but I was so afraid. I was fearful that changing my intensity was a slippery slope into deconditioning, gaining weight, and my POTS symptoms getting worse. My doctor had told me that if I had not already been so physically fit when my POTS began, I might have been bedridden by now. Fortunately, I did eventually change things up by eliminating the intense cardio workouts and adding in more yoga and weights. I was actually able to maintain my weight, without becoming a drunken sloth after each workout.

Many other seemingly simple changes were incredibly tough for me to implement, and took even longer to accept and embrace. Learning to pace myself, to give things up, to ask for help and to not care what others think were some of my hardest lessons to learn. In fact, I am still learning them now. I was always someone who pushed through to get everything done and couldn't enjoy myself until all my work was finished. Even if a package arrived that I had waited a long time for and couldn't wait to open, I would refuse to touch it till all my tasks were completed and I could sit down and thoroughly enjoy what was inside. I suppose many would consider this a strength, but in many ways—even before POTS—it was a huge downfall for me.

Think about being the mother of three small children combined with that drive to get everything done before taking the time to enjoy anything. It just doesn't serve you well. I took the time to spend with my kids and play with them, but I was always worried about all the things that I still needed to get done. And, as I had done earlier in life, I worried about whatever it was I *wasn't* doing. When I was getting things done, I felt guilty and sad that I wasn't spending time with the kids. When I was spending time with them, I was still caught up worrying about getting things done.

Then POTS entered the picture, and I fought *so* hard to keep doing it all. I knew that I should be pacing myself, but I didn't want to be weak. At least that is how I viewed slowing down at the time. Dr. Sica had advised that a balance was crucial—too much activity and I'd make myself worse, yet too little activity was "the kiss of death," as he put it. I was certainly finding this to be true on my own. I knew he was right, but it takes a lot more than head knowledge to change years of learned behavior and personality traits.

And yes, I didn't just say behavior, I also said personality.

I know that we tend to think utopian ideas like, "I'd never let (insert greatest trial you are facing) change me." But the fact is, our trials *do* change us. Honestly, it would be a pretty sad waste of our pain if they didn't. We can continue to insist that we will stay the same. However, then we tend to become bitter and angry at our situation. We invest all our energy in "if only's." Change has still happened, but unfortunately, it has turned out to be a negative one. We can sit and throw a pity party that we have to change certain aspects of our life, like my task-minded personality, or we can view change through a different set of lenses. We can choose to believe that change is not only something that we must accept but something that can be embraced because God wants to use our trial to draw us closer to Him and mold our character.

But accepting that God wanted me to change within my trial; that He wanted to trade my brokenness for beauty; that I could, in fact, be better when broken, are things that I have learned to embrace after years with chronic illness. During those earlier years, I was too busy fighting it all.

⟶ ∞∞ ⟵

Even with the correct diagnosis, it was going to take some time to find the right combination of medications and dosages that worked for me. The treatment would not completely cure me—as of now there is no cure for POTS—but would help manage my symptoms to an extent. We went through a lot of trial and error.

Some medications caused pretty awful side effects, so we decided it wasn't worth it to continue; other medications didn't help me at all. I also did my own research and would ask Dr. Sica if he thought specific medications were a good idea for me to try. Again, some options didn't work at all. However, when I suggested Bupropion, Dr. Sica told me, "Well, that typically only works in about a third of POTS patients, but we can give it a try."

Bupropion can increase vasoconstriction and raise blood pressure, and it turned out to be one of my most helpful medications! It is the reason that I can walk up steps again.

I learned that even with the best of doctors, being your own advocate is incredibly important.

It's also important to look for non-medicinal options. I had a friend who had good results with improving some of her health issues by focusing on gut health. She raved about her probiotics and prebiotics and kept encouraging me to try them. I put her off for a long time, but when I finally gave it a try, I discovered that there is a huge connection between our gut and nearly every aspect of our health. Many of my POTS symptoms improved significantly. As awesome as my doctors are, this was something that I would have never learned from them.

However, early on—before we were able to get anywhere close to finding the right combination of medicines or natural supplements—a new problem arose. I was starting to feel really spacey anytime I was sitting, which included driving with my kids in the car, and trying to converse with anyone. It was increasingly difficult to remember what had been said, or worse: I couldn't even remember if a conversation had actually occurred. To be sure the medications weren't causing the issues, I tried stopping the ones I was currently taking, but the problem didn't go away. The only thing that did was exacerbate all my POTS symptoms.

I was also starting to wake up at night—over and over again—because I was dizzy. When I told Greg and Dr. Sica about this, they were both genuinely surprised that the dizziness was significant enough to wake me up. Though it was surprising, it was true: I was woken up, every night, multiple times a night. Dr. Sica wanted me to return to the EP doctor.

As you can imagine, that was about the last thing that I wanted to do. However, he assured me that although he was lacking in bedside manner, the EP doc was the best person to see in this situation. "Besides, I'm going to call him myself and tell him exactly what I want him to do for you." Then he picked up the phone and called him on the spot! Unfortunately, there was no answer, but Dr. Sica assured me that he would speak with him personally before my appointment.

When I arrived for my visit, the EP doc was much friendlier this time around. Perhaps Dr. Sica changed his mind about me—or maybe he was just having a better day himself—but for whatever reason, he seemed willing to run the test that Dr. Sica wanted: a 30-day event monitor. Yuck. I had been down this road before. Although I had started taking my heart rate during some of these spacey incidents, finding it to be in the 40s, I didn't think they were going to find anything that would affect our treatment. However, I wanted to do what Dr. Sica wanted and not irritate the EP doc.

While wearing the monitor, the same issues continued throughout the following 30 days. The dizziness woke me up many times a night, and the spaciness only seemed to increase.

Soon after starting, the people from the monitoring company called me, "Are you alright, Mrs. Maddox?"

"I'm fine. Why would you call to ask that?"

"We just wanted to make sure; your heart rate is dropping very low."

Oh boy. That couldn't be a good sign. I had a feeling that I wasn't going to like where this was headed. I called in to the EP doctor's office to ask about the call, and if I should be concerned. The staff took down my message and said they would get back to me. When they returned my call, they said that it wasn't anything to be concerned about. The EP doctor had said that everything was looking normal.

After the way the doctor handled my concern on the phone, Greg decided that he was coming with me to my next appointment. He wanted to be sure I wasn't being brushed off and ensure our questions were answered. When the doctor came in, he began telling us that everything was fine. *Here we go again. What would be the lame excuse now? What? Is my heart rate too low because now I am in too good of shape? Do I need to exercise less? Had he even looked at any of the reports from my 30-day monitor?*

Fortunately, he then turned to his computer and pulled up the results ... and suddenly changed his tune. Too much, actually. Now I *didn't* want this much concern from him, and he was the one frustrated with us because we weren't giving him any answers regarding the treatment options he was throwing out. The truth was, we needed some time to process all that he was suggesting.

A pacemaker. At 35 years old? Although he didn't strike me as someone who spent much time engaging in humor, I was still convinced he had to be joking.

Well, he wasn't joking, but what he was suggesting was a bit unconventional. Since I was so young, and I didn't have a life-threatening need for a pacemaker—other than the fact that my low heart rate could have caused a crash while driving, I suppose— he wanted to put in what he called "a temporary permanent pacemaker." I couldn't figure that one out. I mean, wasn't that the definition of an oxymoron? It didn't make any sense to me, but eventually, after many calls and questions, I understood.

He wanted to put a pacemaker (that was meant to be permanent) on the *outside* of my body, literally taped to my chest, with a wire that ran from it into my neck and down into my heart. Therefore, since the pacemaker itself was not implanted in my body, it could be removed somewhat simply and was considered temporary. The idea was new. So new, in fact, that no cardiologist I talked to had ever heard of it. The purpose was to determine if it made a significant enough difference for me to warrant implanting a permanent pacemaker. I still wasn't 100% sure about it, but after continuing to feel unsafe while driving and not being able to sleep, we decided to give it a try.

Fortunately, it was winter; otherwise, it would have been incredibly hard to hide a wire coming out of my neck and a pacemaker taped to my chest. However, it was still tricky to try to cover up. Who would have imagined a year before that I'd be borrowing turtlenecks from my grandma to hide my pacemaker! Plus, wearing high turtlenecks to work in a hospital where you're on the go all day gets pretty hot.

A couple days after I had the temporary pacemaker put in, my cousin, Joanne, and my friend, Lacey, showed up at church with unexpected gifts for me.

Feeling surprised and slightly confused, I asked, "What are these for?"

"Just open them, you'll see."

It took everything in me to not burst into tears immediately when I pulled out two infinity scarves. It was such a simple gift, but it was so thoughtful. They knew it was going to be a struggle to keep this device hidden, and they knew I was self-conscious about it. I can't put into words what that meant to me. My heart is warmed every time I wear them—even now.

Never underestimate the impact your simple acts of kindness have on friends and family when they are in the midst of heartache or vulnerable times in their lives. Sometimes all it takes is a scarf to get you through some extraordinarily dark days.

With my turtlenecks and scarves, I was all set to spend the next few weeks with a device meant for the elderly taped to my 35-year-old chest. A pacemaker keeps your heart rate from dropping too low. So, the doctor can set whatever rate he would like you to stay above. The first week, the doctors set the pacemaker but didn't tell me what rate they were setting it to. They wanted me to keep track of all the symptoms I was experiencing, and when I returned a week later, they'd have me report any changes, good or bad. Then they changed the settings on the pacemaker—again not telling me what they were doing—and we would repeat the cycle. I suppose it was meant to be a single-blind study, but it doesn't take a rocket scientist to tell when your heart rate is dropping to the 30s and 40s and when it's not.

After the first week of the pacemaker being set to keep me from dropping below 60 beats per minute, I felt *so* much better. I was sleeping more regularly, was more alert and felt less spacey when sitting, and could think more clearly. When they turned it off, I could tell before I even checked my heart rate. I felt like a space cadet again, and I'd start waking up from dizziness. That was all the doctor needed.

"Alright, let's go ahead and schedule your permanent pacemaker."

"Wait a minute. I know that this helped, but I need to be convinced beyond a shadow of a doubt before I let you put a pacemaker in my 35-year-old body. Can't we stick with the temporary one a little longer? Can't you keep changing the settings so I can see if my symptoms stay consistent with how it's set?"

This time he was exceptionally kind, "I think we can do that. We can't leave this temporary one in forever due to the risk of infection, you know. But we can afford to keep it there for a couple more weeks if that is what you need to be sure about this decision."

It was what I needed. And it did convince me.

We set up my permanent pacemaker to be implanted on March 6, 2014. Greg and I were heading to the beach *alone* on March 16, so that would give me plenty of time to recuperate. As utterly exhausted parents with lots going on, we were desperately looking forward to that trip. I knew I wouldn't be able to enjoy the hot tub, but at least I wouldn't have this wire and crazy device to hide. I was looking forward to Greg and I rollerblading on the boardwalk to the sound of the crashing waves. This whole ordeal would be behind us.

March 6 came and went uneventfully. The only unexpected thing was that they asked if I'd like to be part of a research study on an MRI compatible pacemaker. They thought I'd be a good candidate for the study since I was so young and would likely need an MRI at some point in my lifetime. I was very pleased with this. Due to my ever-changing health issues, not being able to have MRIs was one thing that had concerned me about getting a pacemaker. As part of the research study, I would have a couple of additional appointments and would possibly have an MRI a few months after the pacemaker was placed, but I was more than willing to do it.

After the surgery, I was on bedrest for several hours but was able to leave the next morning. And as a side note, I think every healthcare worker should be forced to use a bedpan at least once in their life; maybe then we'd all have a lot more compassion and get our patients to an actual toilet or bedside commode whenever possible!

During my first night at home, every time I turned over in bed or tried to get comfortable, I would have pain in my chest. I thought it was a bit odd, but was too exhausted to care too much. In the morning when I sat up on the edge of the bed, the pain in my chest suddenly intensified. I was a little confused because I have seen many elderly people after they have gotten their pacemakers, and I've never heard anyone complain of chest pain.

I looked over the post-op instructions but didn't see chest pain listed as something to call about. I suppose I should have done so anyway, but I guess I wasn't thinking clearly and just brushed it off. I thought, *Well, surely some chest pain is normal. After all, Dr. Sica said that POTS would make any other underlying condition worse. I'm probably just going to experience things a little more intensely.* So, I took one of the pain medications that I had been prescribed, and I went with my family to church.

That's what normal people do when they are having chest pain after a surgery, right? I was careful. I even wore the sling they gave me so people wouldn't forget and hug me too tight.

Throughout the next couple of days, the pain continued to intensify—sometimes spreading up into my throat and jaw—but then it started to slack off. *See*, I thought, *It was just me and my weird medical issues causing me to take a little longer to recover than normal.*

On Friday afternoon, eight days after the surgery, I texted my sister, Kimi, who had been quite worried about me, telling her that I was fine. I told her that everything was pretty much back to normal. I had even gone for a walk/jog that day, as I was still jogging at this point in time. I hadn't learned to give it up yet. I had taken it easy since it was my first time exercising again since surgery, but overall, I felt pretty good.

That night I rolled over in bed, and the same familiar pain in my chest was back—only this time, it was more intense. *Don't tell me I irritated something with my jog.* It took me a while to find a comfortable position. Simply getting used to a metal device in your chest takes some new positioning at first, but I was able to get back to sleep. When I sat up the next morning, the pain that hit me took my breath away. It was not only in my chest, but was also pulsating up into my neck and throat. I didn't know what to do.

It was Saturday, so Greg was there. Always the early riser, he was already up and out in the kitchen. It's not like I didn't have anyone to help, but Saturday is the Sabbath. It's the day we go to church, and I was supposed to teach the children's Sabbath school class (which is essentially Sunday school on Saturday).

I take my commitments very seriously.

I decided to take some of the pain medication that they had given me after surgery, and still, I struggled through getting ready for church. When I drug myself out to the kitchen, Greg immediately knew that something was wrong.

"I need to take you to the hospital."

"No, you don't. This is the same kind of pain that I had before, and it went away. I just aggravated it again by running yesterday. It will settle down in a little bit."

Greg kept arguing with me, but eventually gave up because he knows it's pointless when my mind is made up. Looking back, I realize I'm a lot like some of those stubborn little old men at work who I shake my head at; the ones who wait days before coming to the hospital, making their condition much worse than it would have been if they had just come in the first place.

We went to church, and it was hard to even make it down the stairs to the room where I taught my class. Greg kept arguing with me before it started, and finally said, "Okay, as soon as this is over, I'm taking you to the hospital."

I looked him dead in the eye and said, "The only place I am going is to the beach. With you. Tomorrow." Hmmm ... little old man.

During the class, when a child dropped a felt piece on the floor, or items needed to be collected, I realized I couldn't bend over to get them. If I did, the throbbing became so intense that I was afraid I'd yell out in pain. I started to point to the items for Greg to pick them up. "Why can't *you* pick it up?" he wanted to know.

After class, Greg was insistent, "If your pain is getting worse when you bend over, then I'm afraid the wire has damaged your heart. You could be bleeding into your pericardium! I'm taking you to the hospital!"

"You are a paranoid husband. You are taking me to the beach ... tomorrow."

Greg didn't think I was funny or cute by this point. He meant business.

"Okay." I caved. "If the pain isn't any better by the time church is over, then you can take me to the hospital."

By the time church ended, I was a more than willing patient. I could barely make it to the car.

The hospital where all my doctors are located is an hour away. By the time we got there, I couldn't even walk into the emergency room from the curb without stopping to rest. When I finally made it to the counter I was so short of breath that I could barely get out, "I'm having chest pain ... I got a pacemaker last week."

The woman at the counter directed me to the waiting room, which was packed. Greg had been parking the car, and when he came in, he couldn't believe I was sitting in the waiting room. "When you come in with chest pain that intense you should be taken straight back!"

"Well, the waiting room is full."

"That doesn't even matter!"

He turned around, ready to make some heads roll. Fortunately for them, they came out and called my name. When I stood up, I could see the bewildered and frustrated looks on the faces of the people who had been waiting for who knows how many hours. I had just come in and looked perfectly young and healthy, yet I was called back within a few minutes.

They performed an electrocardiogram, which was normal. Then they moved me to one of the rooms in the emergency department. They did a chest X-ray, which looked fine. They could see the pacemaker, and it appeared to be just as it was when I left this same hospital eight days ago. No one seemed terribly concerned until they brought in the machine that interrogates my pacemaker and found that one of the wires was requiring much more energy than it had been before.

I could tell from the look on Greg's face that he knew what that meant, but I didn't.

"Well, what does that mean?" I asked the doctor while thinking, *That better not mean the battery is going to run out faster and I'll need to have it replaced quicker.*

"It means that we are going to have to admit you and fix it."

"Like, today?!"

"Yes, today. Well, we will admit you today, but we won't be able to do the surgery to fix your wire until Monday. You want that to be done when all the usual staff that performs these procedures are here, so it will wait till Monday."

"And then I go home Monday?"

"No. You will need to stay overnight after the surgery."

"So I will go home Tuesday."

"At the earliest."

" ... I'm supposed to go to the beach tomorrow."

I'm sure the doctor couldn't have cared less about that last statement, but honestly, that is all my brain could focus on. While resting on the table, I didn't have any pain, so nothing seemed urgent to me. I don't know if it was shock or denial, but I handled all these interactions like I was talking with my mechanic about whether my car was going to be fixed in time for a road trip. I think perhaps my ridiculous mindset of *beach, beach, beach* was a blessing in disguise. It protected me from any stress, anxiety or panic that could have ensued from what was currently happening and what was about to happen.

"Any chance I can get a private room? We have three young kids, and I know they will want to come see me. They aren't quiet, and I wouldn't want them bothering a roommate."

"We will see. We still need to do an echocardiogram. Hopefully that is fine and doesn't show any fluid surrounding your heart. If it does, you'll be getting a big, private room anyway."

Greg nodded, but I didn't catch what had been implied. I was too busy calculating how many days we would have left at the beach once I got out of there on Tuesday.

When they performed the echocardiogram, Greg was intense as he peered over the doctor's shoulder, looking at the screen showing different images and angles of my heart. I knew something was very important here and that Greg seemed particularly interested in what it may show, but I couldn't quite comprehend what was going on. Then I saw a faint, but sudden look of concern come over Greg's face. I looked at the screen, but it looked the same to me.

The doctor turned to Greg and then pointed at the screen. "Do you see it?"

"Yes, I see it," Greg replied with concern in his voice.

"It's a substantial amount as well."

"What's going on?" Now I knew how my patients must feel when I talk with their family members about them.

The doctor looked me in the eyes and said sympathetically, "It looks like you'll be getting that private room after all."

Being the patient lying in an ICU bed is a very strange experience when you are used to treating patients in the ICU. It seemed surreal that I was there, especially since I felt perfectly fine and normal while lying in bed—with the exception of all the wires and monitors and the draft of air that hit my backside every time I moved.

Before Greg went home that night, he knew I wouldn't ask for the things that would help me sleep, so he told my nurse, "She is going to need some earplugs, lots of blankets, a couple more pillows and an eye mask to shut out the light if you have one. Oh, and please keep the curtain pulled. It helps block the light from the nurses' station."

I had been getting along quite well with my nurse. "High maintenance?" he asked in a high, playful tone.

"Hey, I don't have a catheter, a feeding tube or very many wires. You don't have to bathe me or change my diaper, and I can walk myself to that toilet in the corner. I think you can handle a blanket and a couple pillows!"

He laughed, "Yeah, I think I can handle that."

Just after Greg left, they came and wheeled me down the hall for a chest CT. Since the echocardiogram had shown fluid (that could only be blood) in my pericardium, they needed to be sure that I wasn't actively bleeding or bleeding anywhere else. Fortunately, I wasn't. Having blood in my pericardium was significant enough.

The pericardium is the sack that surrounds the heart; it isn't supposed to have fluid in it, apart from a very small amount for lubrication. If it fills up, it constricts the heart and the heart will have no room to contract and will stop beating. Henceforth, the reason that a perfectly healthy looking 35-year-old was laying in an ICU bed requesting earplugs and eye masks ... and whining about the fact that she is supposed to be going to the beach.

Even with the extra blankets, pillows, earplugs and the makeshift eye mask I whittled out of sheets, sleep was completely elusive. How had I never thought about the fact that the lights never go out in the ICU? All those poor patients. For patients on other floors, they can close their doors and turn off the lights. Yes, they get nurses and aides and lab workers coming in all night, but at least they can have some semblance of darkness for a while. For someone with migraines, the 24/7 fluorescent lights were the hardest part of being in ICU.

It certainly took a toll, because the next day I kept vomiting from a migraine ... even when my kids came to visit. We erroneously thought that if they saw me and realized that I looked perfectly fine, it would ease their worries. But when they arrived, I was having a very hard time. I couldn't stand any noise or them cracking the blinds to peak out the window, and then I started throwing up. I felt terrible, and now they were more worried than ever.

Throughout the rest of the day, there were tons of doctors and residents and students in my room. Groups of them stood outside my door and talked about me, and I could hear the students ooh-ing and ahh-ing. I was a fascinating case. As a healthcare worker, I got that. Everyone wanted in on the action.

The only thing that bothered me was when the residents would talk to each other about me in my room while the doctor was talking to me. It was hard enough to concentrate on what the doctor was saying without hearing other people whispering about you. Especially when they were whispering incorrect assumptions. When they walked in my room, I'd sit up to talk with them. That's all it took for my heart rate to go into the 130s.

The students or residents would all whisper and point at the monitor and say things like, "She's really anxious." Sometimes I wanted to hold a finger up to the doctor talking to me and say, "Could you hold on just a second? This is a teaching moment for your residents." And then I would turn to them and say, "My heart rate went up to 130 not because I am anxious, but because I am sitting. My blood vessels don't constrict when I am upright or standing, so my heart has to pump faster to combat gravity. Now I have a hole in my heart causing bleeding into my pericardium, which doesn't help the situation. You need to do some research on postural orthostatic tachycardia syndrome before you assume anyone is anxious based on heart rate." But I couldn't have told them all of that, because the fast heart rate was making me short of breath ... and also because I didn't have the nerve.

I distinctly remember one visit from the electrophysiologist who did my surgery. This was a different EP doctor than the one I had been seeing. This one was exceptionally kind, with a great bedside manner. He would even call my nurse in the middle of the night while I was in the ICU to see how I was doing. This particular time, he came in with an entourage of four. He told me that in addition to fixing the wire, he was going to do his very best to do my surgery via pericardiocentesis, by wrapping a small tube around my heart that would exit through my abdomen to drain the blood from my pericardium.

For some reason, I had never considered how they would do this. I knew they needed to fix the wire, but hadn't considered how to remove the blood. If that didn't work, then they would need to cut a small hole between my ribs on my left side. Finally, if that didn't work, there was a chance that they would need to go in through my sternum. Because of this chance, they needed to prepare the OR, staffing and me as though we were going into open heart surgery.

"Um, okay. So, if you don't have to do that, do I still get to go home on Tuesday?"

"No. Even if all we do is the tube in your abdomen, you will need to stay until at least Wednesday."

I hadn't batted an eye at the possibility of open heart surgery. But when he told me that I was definitely staying an additional day, I started to cry. I tried hard not to, but I was so exhausted, and the tears had a mind of their own.

"Are you scared?" one of the residents asked gently.

"No. I'm supposed to be at the beach."

On Monday, the day of the surgery, Greg arrived with a bag packed, prepared to stay the night. "That's ridiculous," I scolded. "I don't need you here exhausting yourself. I'm so worn out now, that after anesthesia, I'm sure all I'm going to do is sleep."

"I'm staying. There is no need to discuss it anymore," Greg stated matter-of-factly.

Well, alrighty then. Greg is not typically forceful when we disagree on a decision, so I knew this was important to him.

Greg headed out into the hall to get something and suddenly appeared around the curtain again, "Look who I found!" In walked my brother, Travis, who lives over three hours from the hospital and has a job that does not involve having Mondays off. I couldn't believe that he had come.

"Where else did you think I would be?" he said.

Before long, my parents arrived. I knew they were exhausted because they had been taking care of *someone's* unruly children since Saturday, yet, they had gotten a friend to watch the kids so they could be there. I'm sure my sisters would have been there as well if it had not required airline tickets and extensive childcare hoops to make it happen, and I'm certain my in-laws would have been right by our sides if they had not been out of the country.

Throughout the hospital stay, we had so many visits, phone calls and texts. The support of family and friends meant so much to us.

I don't remember a lot about the time just before surgery, apart from my mom seeming very scared and that the bed that they were taking me to the operating room on had power assist. The motor was out of control, and it was going too fast; the nurses kept crashing it into the walls. I felt bad for them knowing how stressful it is to be on their end, trying to protect your patient and her family and not cause any damage. But from my end, it was pretty darn funny.

When I woke up, it was similar to when I woke from my endometriosis surgery. I was awake for a long time, but couldn't move or open my eyes.

That is where the similarities ended though, because I was also in excruciating pain.

Why was I in such intense pain? No one prepared me for this! To me, that could only mean one thing. *They've cracked my chest!* As soon as I could move, I started trying to get my hand up to my chest, trying to see if it was bandaged. Greg would take my hand and lay it back down and say, "Just rest now, Cristy." I'd try again, and he would do the same. It was maddening. I couldn't ask what was going on and he wasn't telling me.

Finally, the anesthesia wore off enough that I was able to ask, "What happened?"

"You had surgery to repair your pacemaker. You're okay, just rest."

Well, duh! I knew that much!

Eventually, I was able to ask, "Did I have open heart?"

"Oh no! No, no. They were able to do everything with just the tube in your abdomen."

I was relieved, but still confused. "Then why am I in so much pain?"

"Is it bad?"

I nodded. "It might be worse than childbirth."

Greg turned around and headed straight out the door to find the nurse, who returned and gave me two milligrams of Dilaudid through my IV. I immediately felt better, but five minutes later the pain was back at full intensity. They gave me two more milligrams with the same results. When the pain returned, Greg headed out again. He came back in just a minute and said, "They are getting you a pain pump."

Later I asked him if they were already planning on that or if he had insisted. He said he told the resident that I was very tough with pain, had given birth naturally and had said this was possibly worse than childbirth. Then he told them, "She needs a pain pump. There is no way your nurse is going to be able to keep up with her." They didn't argue.

Once I had the pain pump, I felt so much better. Even though I was shocked by the amount of pain I was having after this surgery, apparently Greg was not. Now I understood why he was so insistent on staying the night with me, and I was so thankful he had. I would have been terrified that night without him.

The next day, Greg asked me, "Do you have any idea how much blood drained from your pericardium?"

"No clue."

"300 mL!"

"Okay. I still have no clue what that means." I didn't know how much was supposed to be in there to begin with, so that meant nothing to me.

Everyone else seemed completely shocked, however. When I finally returned to work, even Dr. Agyeman came up to me and said, "Okay, your coworkers told me what happened and how much blood they drained, but I don't believe it. I need to hear it from you."

When I told him, he still didn't seem to believe my story. "You don't understand," he said. "That never happens. That's the kind of thing that they put on the medical boards that annoys medical students because you know that you will *never* actually see it. But they put it on there because it is within the realm of possibility."

The pericardium typically only has 5-10 milliliters of fluid in it, but up to 50 mL is normal. It can hold 80-200mL of fluid that develops acutely, and as much as 2 liters (2000 mL) if the fluid accumulates very slowly over time. I had 300 mL in mine, so even though some had happened fairly quickly after my jog, obviously some had been developing for a while.

With the blood drained, my pain was much improved, and I didn't need the pain pump anymore, but I was very lethargic. I couldn't focus or stay awake. I had been ridiculously nauseated and had hardly eaten anything, so when they brought my lunch, I *tried* to eat something but kept falling asleep with the fork in my hand. It now made sense why they weren't going to let me leave the day after my surgery.

A nurse came in and removed the intermittent compression device that squeezed my calves to keep my blood circulating. It was strange that after all that had happened, that was the most surreal moment of the entire hospital stay for me because I have removed those on patients of mine hundreds—if not thousands—of times. That was the moment when I felt like the reality finally hit me, *Oh my word! This is happening to me.*

I had been in ICU for three days, had a wire in my heart repaired, and a tube wrapped around my heart and coming out of my abdomen, but it was a nurse un-Velcroing cloth cuffs from my legs that made the reality sink in. When I tried to get up to the bathroom, I was floored by how weak I was. When I made a remark to this effect, the nurse said, "That is to be expected. Being in bed for several days will make you weak, even if you are perfectly healthy. Your body has been through a lot of trauma, so it is going to take you a little while to regain your strength."

I almost laughed at her. I wanted to say, "Wait a second! *I* am the one who usually gets patients up and gives them that talk!" It's funny how I could give that talk to others, believe it 100% to be true, yet be completely shocked when it actually happened to me.

The doctors seemed pleased, though. They performed my sixth and seventh echocardiograms that day. They were serious about watching how much fluid was surrounding my heart. I had two echocardiograms a day, performed in my room by a doctor. I should have known, but the significance of this did not dawn on me till I was out of the woods and all I needed was one more echocardiogram before I could be discharged home.

I thought it would be simple. Just send in the doctor with the machine again! However, it seemed to take an eternity because I had to wait for transport to come and take me to the cardiovascular lab, then wait there for someone I'd never seen before to do the test, then wait for transport to come again to return me to my room and then wait for the doctor to look at the results.

I guess when the blood drained from my pericardium, I lost my VIP status.

───

We were finally able to leave around noon on Wednesday, and yes, you guessed it: we went to the beach. It was not at all the experience we had anticipated, and it was significantly abbreviated, but we were very thankful that we still were able to have a couple of nights there. Besides, I needed it. I was in no shape at that point to return home and try to take care of the kids, so in that respect, it had been good timing.

I don't know if things would have been any better if I had gone to the doctor as soon as I started having pain in my chest. It seemed something wasn't right with that wire from my first night home, and I was probably bleeding into my pericardium all along.

However, I kept pushing through. It's what a mom is supposed to do, right?

What I do know is that I was in a life-threatening situation and I didn't consider the possibility that my physical needs trumped my responsibilities at church that day. My responsibilities as a mother should have sent me running straight for the emergency room. How could I risk what my children would go through if something happened to me, simply because I didn't know how to give things up; to let people down? This was such a hard-fought lesson for me to learn, and I nearly paid for it with my life.

I'd like to say that after this, the lesson was seared into my very soul. I wish I could report that from then on, I put my health and therefore my family at the top of my to-do list.

But did I mention that I am hard-headed?

They found a hole in my heart, but they probably should have checked my head as well.

CHAPTER FOUR

I Don't Need Help

"Can prayer change our circumstances? Absolutely!
But when our circumstances don't change,
it's often an indication that
God is trying to change us."
— Mark Batterson, Draw the Circle

What is that they say? Pride goeth before a fall? Well, sometimes pride goeth during and after a fall as well.

Every summer for as long as I can remember, our family attended camp meeting. Camp meeting is essentially Vacation Bible School for all ages, and people come from all over Virginia and Maryland to attend.

That particular morning wasn't terribly hot; 80 degrees at most. All five of us were rushing around in our 14'x14' cinder block room that served as bedroom and kitchen. One double bunk and a three-high bunk bed stood in the corner. A curtain divided the beds from the dorm-sized refrigerator, toaster oven and small table.

As the kids finished breakfast, we dumped their paper plates and plastic forks in the trash. There was no way I was going to attempt dishes without a sink. As I handed the kids their toothbrushes and toothpaste, we hurried them out the door and another 150 feet down the row of cinder block rooms to the bathroom to wash up.

"You better hurry up if you don't want to miss the songs!" I called out after them.

After a couple of minutes, Aiden returned. He was always diligent about being on time. Anxious to head out, he put his things away, grabbed his Bible and hurried off to his class.

Looking out the door to check on the younger two, I sighed. As I suspected, they had gotten distracted and were playing ball with some kids in the grass between the rows of rooms. Carrington's toothbrush lay in the grass.

I was frustrated, but really couldn't blame them—this was heaven to a couple of country kids. When they walk out their door at home, they're not going to see another child unless we get in the car and drive several miles. However, this place was different. Here at camp meeting, you can't even go to the bathroom without running into ten other kids. This was a dream come true for them.

—☙✦☙—

It was a dream for me as well—I loved coming to camp as a kid. I looked forward to it every summer. Back then, we would pack seven of us into an identical 14'x14' "cabin." If you could believe it, my mom actually washed the dishes *without* a sink! In my young, impressionable mind, the word cabin simply meant a 14'x14' cinder block room. Looking back, I'm not sure why we called them that since cabin sounds far too luxurious.

Regardless of the terminology, I loved those cinder block rooms because it meant that we were surrounded by other children. Being a country kid myself, I treasured the times I was able to interact and play with kids right outside my door. I looked forward to the classes that were put on by our church; there were several per day for every age group. A week full of songs, crafts, activities and learning more about Jesus. And kids! So much fun with other kids. What could possibly be better?

As an adult, I still loved spending time at camp meeting.

Honestly, now that I think about it, I'm not sure why—especially as a parent. You spend days packing everything under the sun from curtains, to cleaning supplies, a toaster oven and an a/c unit. After you finally arrive, you then spend all your time trying to corral your kids, get them fed and clean without a stove or running water, and keep them quiet in class. We never made it to any classes for the adults; we were too exhausted.

Despite the rigorous preparation, lack of amenities and complete exhaustion, I loved that my kids were able to have the same experience that I had as a child. I loved that they were learning more about Jesus, and I loved seeing their joy—but it was so much more than that.

Unfortunately, the "more" did not involve any sort of spiritual experience. It was more of an "I am woman, hear me roar" type of feeling. I can handle taking care of all these cranky kids in this environment and keep up with running them all over creation. I can do it all.

And I mean, *check us out*. We can rough it. I know it's not exactly camping, but hey, we proved that we could live with hardly anything—and like it too! We are not *that* spoiled. Well, I knew we were spoiled in the sense that nearly all Americans are spoiled. But it made me feel that I was not as absorbed in the consumerism mindset that is so prevalent in our culture today. I guess I had something to prove ... which probably meant there was a bigger issue in the first place.

—⚬⚬⚬—

"Get your toothbrush out of the grass!" I called to Carrington, making sure she knew she and Noah needed to put their things away. It was time for class. As they finished cleaning up, Greg started to hurry them out the door. "Wait for me!" I yelled after them. Surprised, he turned around and replied, "You're coming? You don't have to do that, you know."

"I know," I answered. "But I want to. Camp meeting is halfway over already, and I haven't even been up the hill to their classes yet. I want to be able to peek in at them at least once and see what they're doing."

"Okay. Do you want me to go get the van?"

"No. I'm feeling okay, and it's not that hot. I'll just take it slow."

It was a beautiful day, and even though I was feeling perfectly fine, we took our time. "Wait for Mama!" Greg called after the kids, as we slowed our steps to a snail's pace on the way up the hill.

Wait for Mama. How many times had they heard that called to them over the last couple of years? When did *their* freedom become so limited because of *me*? As a mother, that was the most difficult aspect of this challenge; how it affected my children.

The peacefulness and beauty of the day were starkly contrasted by the chaos that met us the moment we opened the door to the school where the classes were held. So many people, and so much *noise*.

But we've learned to deal. Greg automatically gave me his left arm, knowing I'd start to lose my balance toward my right side. We took Noah to his class and Carrington to hers. I watched each of them through the doors for a few minutes. I was proud of Carrington's confidence as she strode into class and how Noah was making friends and singing along with the songs. Even with the noise, I was happy I had come.

We bumped into a couple old friends and talked for a few minutes. It was warm in the building, and of course, there was nowhere to sit. However, I hated to pass up an opportunity to talk with people. I hadn't seen many of the people I usually got to see because I was spending so much time in our *luxury cabin*.

Sometimes when I did see someone at the bathrooms, they'd be surprised and say something like, "I didn't even know you were here this year. I've seen Greg every day, but I haven't seen you. You look great!" I had just gone from a size twelve to a size eight in a six-week period—and the pounds were still melting away. All my life I'd tried to lose weight. But now, all I wanted to do was be able to eat without suffering the consequences.

When we finished visiting, I told Greg firmly, "I need to get out of here." The noise, warmth and motion were beginning to take a toll, but once I made it outside, I felt better. There was hardly anyone around when classes were in session, so it was very quiet.

After a couple minutes away from the commotion, I didn't need his arm for support anymore, and we walked hand in hand down the hill. The distance to the cabin is not very far, and since it was downhill this time, I didn't give it much thought. However, we'd only gone about half the distance when my right leg started to feel weak. Not unusual. "I'll make it," I thought.

Unfortunately, within another 50 feet, I could barely pull my right leg forward anymore, and my right hand was beginning to tremor. We were in the middle of an open field of grass with no shade anywhere, so stopping was not an option. I had to get out of the heat.

Greg began asking me if I was okay. One of the most difficult parts of this whole ordeal is that when I really need to tell him what's going on, I simply can't. There was no way I could attempt to formulate an answer and try to get my leg to work at the same time. Wasn't happening. So, I kept pushing forward, ignoring Greg's questions and attempts to help. I was focused on one small area of shade on the concrete next to the men's bathroom.

It took all my energy, but I made it. I thought that if I could just stand in the shade to rest, then I would be able to make it the rest of the way—I didn't want to sit down and have to get back up again. But, by the time I finally got there, I just about collapsed on the ground.

Fortunately, Greg understood and helped lower me as I unsuccessfully tried to catch my breath. He handed me a water bottle after I had made it safely to the ground, and even though I wanted a drink, air was too important at the moment. He was asking me if he should go find a golf cart. The campus that camp meeting is held at is quite large, and many of the pastors drive golf carts around to help transport people from place to place.

"No way," I answered. At least that is what I thought I did. There were a lot of things that I *thought* I told him during that time. However, he later informed me that I never said a word. The

I Don't Need Help

last thing I wanted was for anyone to see what was happening; much less have to ask for help.

"I'll just rest here for a minute, and then I'll be able to make it back," I told him, but apparently the words were only spoken in my mind. I kept resting, and although my breathing subsided enough to drink, I still couldn't get up. Every time I moved my head, the world moved with it. I'm still not sure exactly how long I sat there "talking" to Greg about what to do.

Eventually, a golf cart rounded the corner with two pastors riding in it. They stopped and asked if we needed help. "Nope. We don't," I said while thinking, *What will we do if they don't help?*

Fortunately, they didn't hear me, because apparently, I was never speaking anyway.

Greg told them we needed some assistance to get me to our cabin. Greg helped me up, and he and one of the pastors helped (maybe more like carried) me to the cart. I felt pretty ridiculous when Greg directed them to our cabin, which was just 150 feet away. As they guided me inside, they asked if they should call for first aid or an ambulance. Greg reassured them that that was not necessary.

"It's a chronic medical condition. She'll be alright once she rests in the a/c."

He was right. There was no permanent damage.

Except for my pride.

⸺⸺⸺

After enduring situations like the incident at camp meeting and my pacemaker drama, I continued to push through and do everything I possibly could on my own. Why? Well, because of pride and a fear of asking others for help. And also, because, at least for me, sometimes one of the hardest things in life is mustering the strength to succumb to weakness. We live in a society of fixers, doers and achievers. We value hard work and putting up a good fight. It is a beautiful thing to see an injured athlete limp across a finish line long after the rest have completed the race. It is admirable when someone with a terminal illness fights for as long as they can, against all odds, with every means possible.

We root for the underdog. Who doesn't love a comeback story? You know, the weak becomes strong, rags to riches journey. It is deeply ingrained in our hearts and our culture.

However, for many of us, there are certain times and situations when we must step back, take a long hard look at ourselves and realize that our strength has become our greatest weakness. We must recognize that in order to be strong again, we must admit—and yes, even *give in*—to our weakness.

It almost sounds sacrilegious, I know.

Yet, there are plenty of instances of a supposed strength easily becoming a weakness. Take men for example. They are fixers. It is a great quality, but if the woman in their life has a problem, they want to swoop in and solve it. However, the woman often doesn't even want them to fix it. She doesn't want or need a strong hero to save the day. She wants a friend who listens.

But by using his strength of fixing things, he unknowingly negates her feelings and does not provide what she needs. If the problems are big, he can also feel insecure if he cannot find a solution to them, or feel disrespected that she isn't following his suggestions. Sometimes he feels frustrated and out of control, and is more likely to try to exert his authority in other areas of his life. Over time, their relationship can become damaged and weak. It is better if he admits that he cannot fix it, or better yet, recognizes that it is not his job to solve all of her problems. It is better to realize that to try would only turn one of his strongest qualities into weakness.

Most women are more emotional than men. This is a strength because it helps us connect with each other and our children in wonderful ways. However, it can also prevent us from looking objectively or fairly on interactions with the man in our life. We expect our strength to also be his, which leads to unrealistic expectations and disappointment. If we can admit to this weakness of ours—letting our emotions get in the way—and look at problems that arise more objectively, (dare I say logically), it would bring tremendous gain. Our expectations would be more realistic, our disappointments fewer and our overall contentment higher. Again, a strength can become a weakness.

But those are some obvious examples. What I am really referring to is the tension between our culture idolizing strength and productivity vs. unique life situations that can arise. Situations that create a new weakness, whether acute or chronic, social, financial, physical, mental or spiritual. Situations like ... I don't know ... say, POTS.

My chronic illness came on slowly over time. Fortunately, it did not hit all at once; I wasn't immediately dealing with the quantity and intensity of symptoms that I now have. It has been nearly a decade since the onset, and the gradual progress allowed us to adjust slowly.

But it also caused me to keep pushing hard. Too hard.

This tension played out much like the onset of a cold. You don't feel well, but life is busy, so you power through. However, it doesn't go away. Instead, it gets worse and worse, but you think it will eventually get better so you keep pushing forward until one day you end up in the hospital with pneumonia. You thought you were being strong, taking care of your family and responsibilities, but in reality, you were delaying the care you needed and making yourself worse.

With each new symptom or worsening of a current one, I was sure it was temporary. So, I kept telling myself just to keep pushing. Just a little longer. Just make it through the day, the afternoon, the next five minutes. After a while, pushing through while feeling awful became the new normal. Even though I was absolutely miserable and getting worse all the time, I couldn't bring myself to ask anyone for help. After all, I'd managed to get by this long, so why should I suddenly need help now?

Besides, there were so many other people who needed help much more than we did. Why should I be the one to receive help? I mean, it wasn't like I was going through cancer treatment or dealing with a terminal illness. And how do you ask for help when the help you need isn't just for a season? We couldn't say, "We just need someone to fill in till this treatment is done." People had their own busy lives, and this wasn't temporary. It would require us asking for help over and over and over again, and that just seemed more stressful and exhausting to me than powering through. It wasn't something that I was capable of or ready to do.

This was our life now, so at the time it felt like asking for help would be an exercise in futility.

In this new life, no matter how hard I pushed, things had to slowly start going by the wayside, one by one. Everything that could be put on the back burner was eventually placed there. The house was both messy and dirty; the flower beds full of weeds and the drawers and closets a jumbled mess. Everything left seemed essential. The kids needed to be fed (and they were not getting nice meals, that's for sure). They had to be educated and clothed. And I did still have to go to work, even if it was only one or two days a week.

The only non-essential I had left was teaching the children's class at church, but I couldn't bring myself to tell the church that I couldn't do it anymore. I couldn't stand the thought of letting other people down. They didn't have much help, and after all, two of the kids in the class were mine! I didn't know who else they could get to teach, so I struggled through it week after week.

It became my most dreaded task. My adrenaline would shoot up so high that my already elevated heart rate was nearly intolerable. My hands would be trembling, my legs felt like noodles, and I was dizzy. Yet I still had to sing songs, hand out felts and try to remember stories while telling them to wiggling, noisy children who didn't want to stay in their seats. If a visitor walked in, it was hard not to burst into tears.

I began to dread not only teaching the class, but going to church altogether because of the intense stress and complete and utter exhaustion it would bring.

I hated the loss of a sense of control that I felt when my adrenaline would surge and my heart rate would rise. This was not a normal, I'm-feeling-stage-fright kind of adrenaline; although, even that would have been a little odd since I'd taught this class for a long time. This was an, "I've-narrowly-missed-being-hit-by-an-18-wheeler-while-crossing-the-street kind of adrenaline." The kind that makes you want to crumple to the ground and catch your breath for several minutes.

Yet there were many times when kind church members would poke their head in the room and ask if I needed anything. I'd smile sweetly and say, "No, I don't think so." When really, I wanted to say, "Yeah, could you just take these felts and teach this class for the next five years?"

And I hated that I hated it so much. I had been teaching this class for several years. Why did it have to be such a big deal? I should be happy when visitors came. I caught myself sometimes praying before class that no visitors would show up, and I felt like the world's biggest hypocrite. Before POTS, I had been all about doing for others, compassion and reaching out. *Here I am Lord, send me.* I couldn't understand people who seemed to do nothing. And now I couldn't even teach a one-hour class, once a week, without hating it.

And I hated who I was becoming.

I thought of the church services that I had done in the past for Compassion International. This was something that I dreamed of doing again once my kids were a little older. Was that all behind me? Was I no longer capable of speaking up for the least of these in this capacity? It made me sad, it made me grieve, and it made me slightly bitter. When I thought of all the people out there doing nothing, having no desire to do anything to help others when they are perfectly capable, my confusion and bitterness increased.

It was clear God had a few more lessons in store for me.

———oroo———

Finally, one night I had a meltdown.

Okay, so "one night" makes it sound like it was a first. It definitely wasn't the first meltdown, or the second, or the twentieth. I could force myself to power through a lot of days, but then by evening, I would completely fall apart. I would just hit a wall (physically *and* emotionally), and my body would not allow me to take another step. My mind could not be rational for another second, and I truly couldn't stand up for a moment longer. It was difficult to find words, and I'd often get angry. Not at the illness. Not at anything rational. It was usually at Greg (lucky him) for not helping me enough in that moment or not recognizing what was happening, or at someone else for something super stupid that made no sense even to me once I was able to lay down a while and restore blood flow to my brain.

This particular night, Greg kneeled by our bed while I laid there and just cried because I couldn't even formulate any words yet. I had not been supine long enough to get sufficient blood back to my brain.

"We have to take something off of you," he said gently. "You can't keep up with all of this."

I nodded my head but thought, *There is nothing left to take off of me.*

Then he continued, "You need to stop teaching Sabbath school. It is time for that to end."

I nodded again. We had discussed this many times before, when I could talk. I always agreed that I needed to quit, but told him that I didn't feel like that was an option because they didn't have anyone else to do it.

It was late, so I went off to sleep for the night, and we didn't discuss it again.

Several days later I was visiting my cousin, Joanne, when she casually says to me, "So I heard that you quit teaching Sabbath school."

You could have picked my jaw up off the floor. "What do you mean?!"

"I mean, that you quit teaching Sabbath school."

"What? Wh ... How? Where did you hear that?"

She said that her stepdad was at the men's prayer group at our church and they were praying about someone to replace me because I had quit.

"Well, why did they think that I quit?!"

"Because you sent an email to the elders letting them know that you quit."

"No, I did not!!"

The night after my meltdown, after I fell asleep, Greg had gone and sent an email to my dad (who was head elder) and a couple other church leaders telling them that I quit. He even gave a date of what my last day would be—just two weeks later.

At first, I was mad at him. He had no right! It was not his place, and I asked him why he would do such a thing. He was shocked that I was upset.

"Because the other night you agreed that it was time to quit, but you needed to go to sleep, so I sent the message for you."

In his man-mind, that was all there was to it. We had a problem. I agreed to the obvious solution. He fixed it. So, why did we have a problem now? (And just to be clear, he did not send it from my email. It was from his own account, and it was signed by him.)

After I cooled my jets a bit, relief flooded over me. I was done teaching the class! Only a couple more weeks to go. After those weeks passed, I could not believe how happy I felt again on Sabbath morning. My weekend started on Friday night again rather than after church on Saturday (which didn't leave much weekend when I worked on Sunday). I actually began to look forward to church again.

Greg had done something for me that I was incapable of doing for myself at that time: asking for help and beginning the process of admitting the full extent of my weakness.

Yeah, I realize that this kinda contradicts my earlier example of men trying to fix stuff they shouldn't. Give me a break; I've got POTS brain.

However, this was something that I truly needed to be fixed. I needed the church to help me by finding someone else to teach. I needed to be willing to let people down, which was exactly what I felt like I was doing. I needed my church family and those I loved to know just how bad things were getting. We needed to *not* go this alone any longer.

My hard work ethic? That power through mentality? It had helped me accomplish a lot of things in life. It was a strength.

Until it wasn't.

There comes a point in powering through when you realize that you're not fighting the illness—you aren't being brave or admirable—you are hurting yourself, and in the process, you are hurting the people you love the most.

My hard work ethic had become a weakness; it was an enormous stumbling block for me. It blocked my ability to ask for help and get the rest I needed in order to stop making myself worse. It prevented me from living in community, from taking care of my own spiritual needs, and kept me from being the mother that my kids needed and the wife my husband deserved.

What I needed most was to admit and even *succumb* to weakness. Otherwise, I would never get back on the path toward strength.

CHAPTER FIVE

Mommies are Lazy, and Daddies Work Hard

*"I know, O Lord, that Your judgements are
righteous. And that in faithfulness
You have afflicted me."*
— Psalm 119:75, NASB

Admitting weakness, in any capacity, is hard. Not only is it challenging to accept it yourself, but if you're anything like me, it is even harder to show your weakness to those you love most. In any case, choosing to be vulnerable with those closest to you is a great first step to opening yourself up to receive the support you desperately need.

However, there is a big difference between sharing with a few people and putting your weakness on display to be seen by the whole world. At least my friends and relatives knew what lay beneath the facade of my young, healthy-looking body. But strangers had no way of knowing, therefore letting my weakness be seen or needing to reveal it in public brought a whole new level of fear and embarrassment to the surface for me.

Invisible illness is tricky business. Don't get me wrong; I'm glad that I don't look sick. Heck, many people say that I'm looking my best ever, and I can't say that I minded dropping eight pants sizes. But looking healthy makes it intensely awkward when you are in public and you need help. It makes your world ripe for misunderstandings and unsolicited judgement.

———◦◦◦———

Once—just once—at camp meeting, Greg and I decided to attend a meeting for the adults. We wanted to go because Barry Black was speaking. He is the chaplain of the U.S. Senate, and I had recently read one of his books.

Also, his voice sounds exactly like what I am certain the voice of God sounds like. Who would want to miss hearing the voice of God? Not me.

Even if I was feeling okay, I was still nervous about going into that muggy, jam-packed gymnasium. After all, just a couple of days before, I'd ended up on the ground unable to make it to my cabin when I was feeling "fine." The kids were in their classes, so at least we didn't have the wiggles and shakes to contend with. The gym was quite a distance from the cabin, so we rode a golf cart over to the meeting.

We laid out our game plan ahead of time. In the summer, there aren't many places you can go with POTS without having a plan in place. Before the closing prayer, Greg and I would make our exit so that I could avoid walking in the midst of the mass exodus. He could help me out of the gym and onto a golf cart before he headed up the hill to get the kids. The golf cart would deliver me right to the cabin. It should be no big deal.

Even though I hate interrupting a service and drawing any attention to myself, we got up just before closing prayer and made our way to the back of the gym. However, there were a lot of people standing in the aisle who had not found seats, and Barry Black must have set a record that day for the world's fastest public prayer. (Hmm ... I hope that's not why the Senate likes him, feeling as though they can tip their hat to Christianity and get on with their business of wasting time without wasting too much time?) So, by the time we were nearing the back of the gym, the masses were already getting to their feet.

"Hurry," Greg insisted.

I was doing my best, but was experiencing Walmart-phenomenon at a church service, and I hadn't even gotten a great deal on below-average produce. As the crowd was surging behind us, we headed down the steps to where several golf carts were lined up. Greg was holding my arm as I headed around the back of one of the carts to sit behind the driver when a healthy-looking woman about my age approached from the other side. The driver announced to her and the rest of the crowd, "At this point, we are only taking elderly and the handicapped!"

I stopped in my tracks and looked at Greg helplessly. Even though it was evening, it was still hot; I was dizzy, and the cabin was so far away. But, I was neither elderly nor did I *look* handicapped.

In the sternest tone I've ever heard him use with me, Greg insisted, "You get on that cart!" Then he pulled my arm toward the seat I had been headed for. I plopped down behind the driver, and Greg promised he would meet me at the cabin after he got the kids. I felt humiliated, and as elderly and disabled people started to fill up the carts, I felt ashamed that I was taking someone else's spot. What little old lady was going to have to wait in the heat because of me?

I leaned forward and said to the driver, "I know I don't look disabled, but I truly do need to be on this cart." He said okay. However, after dropping everyone else off at their doors or vehicles, he dropped me at the end of the rows of cabins and did not attempt to take me directly to my door. I didn't say anything, as I felt pretty certain that I was okay to go the remaining distance ... but sometimes I wasn't. I never knew. And I was too embarrassed to ask him to take me the rest of the way.

I get it. I don't blame the man. He was rushing back to pick up more people and was trying to transport as many as he possibly could. He didn't know the alter-universe that is POTS. He didn't understand that I truly live in a different world than he does.

In my world, the heat is a dangerous predator that creeps up behind you. Even when you are on the lookout, it will pounce on a single moment of weakness. In my world, the pressure of the atmosphere can alter balance, trigger a migraine, or make the room spin. In my world, I can't tell my kids that I will go do something fun with them ahead of time, because I won't make them promises that I simply don't know if I can keep.

In my world, I had to choose between eating and being able to stay upright, because they both could not happen simultaneously. In my world, every invitation is viewed through the lens of POTS, and accepting takes extensive planning. In my world, energy is like money on a very fixed income; it has to be budgeted as it is in limited supply. I can't run out before the next paycheck, because when it's gone, it's *gone*. In my world, life as I knew it had completely changed ... I had completely changed. I wasn't even sure I knew who I was anymore. Did I, as I knew myself, even exist in this world?

What about my kids' mother? Surely the mother they used to have didn't exist in this world. That was one of the things that I struggled with the most; the fact that my kids didn't seem to remember who I once was. I was the mother who went nonstop from morning till night, accomplishing so much. In this world, all they see is the mom who fatigues quickly, the mom who has to stop and rest all the time, the mom who occasionally tries to play with them, but gets so short of breath that they have to stop the game and wait for her. After all, Noah once said, "Mommies are lazy (he meant tired), and Daddies work hard."

Ouch.

Unfortunately, in this world, they also see the mom who is short-tempered and constantly asking for quiet. In this world, if I did something extra in my day, the kids had to pay the price as well. I may power through the extra work or activity, but in turn, I feel worse in the evening and am too weak to take care of their needs. I'd jump or involuntarily scream at their every noise, and their movements messed with my balance. In this world, chances are, if outsiders happen to see an active, smiling mom during the day, my children will see an unavailable or grumpy, unkind and snappy mom at night.

In my world, I tried not to think about what was happening to us too much; otherwise, grief reigned supreme. Sure, no one had died. But grief applies to so much more than death. In any case, it felt like my old self had been put to death, and I didn't realize how much I loved her till she was gone.

Besides, it didn't seem like the deaths would end. Just as I'd start to get used to a new version of me, something else would start changing, there were new limitations, and I'd find myself trading in the new me for an even newer me. It wasn't easy to be distracted from the losses either; they were with me every moment, every time I stood up, every time I bent over, every time I moved or heard an unexpected noise. Some days were better than others, but the pain of losing who I was never fully left.

As much as I tried not to think about how much my illness was affecting all of our lives, there were times when the weight of it all would hit me like a ton of bricks. Even with all the special challenges in our home on top of my health and physical limitations, nothing crippled me quite like grief. One particular week, the winter before the camp meeting incidents, I was falling apart. I couldn't even begin to talk about it without sobbing, so I wrote:

> This week it was one "small" loss that spiraled me
> downward into grief. We had a warm day. A high of
> 64 degrees in January! The dysautonomia has caused
> small fiber neuropathy, which has caused an inability
> to regulate my body temperature. So, I can't stand to
> go out when it's cold. I wear layers inside all winter,
> and I still feel like I'm freezing. With one warm day
> and baseball season approaching, I was determined to
> go out and throw a ball with my son.
>
> What I didn't figure on was the higher temperature
> causing a drop in atmospheric pressure, which
> triggered faster heart rates and a migraine. By the
> time we finished morning schoolwork, I couldn't
> even glance out the window due to the brightness,

much less go outside. The kids went out. I struggled through laundry and fixing lunch. When I called them in, I collapsed on the couch with sunglasses and noise-canceling headphones, waiting for the Motrin to kick in.

And I was devastated. The one day of the whole winter that I had a chance of going outside with my kids and I couldn't do it. That sorrow just triggered all the emotion that I suppress to keep pushing through each day. I thought of all the ways I am not the mom I used to be; not the person I used to be. All the ways I feel like I fail my kids. I thought of our fourth child that we were never able to adopt, but I still wish for. I thought of how different all of our lives would look if I were well. I was overcome.

But I still had three kids who needed to finish their day's schooling, so I pushed through. Noah was particularly struggling that day in many ways. He couldn't focus. I said, "Buddy, you did so well doing your schoolwork with Daddy the other day. How come you were able to get so much done with him?" With his answer he spoke truth like only a child can, and it was as though all my fears about who I have become as a mother were confirmed.

"Because Daddy's face smiles when he does schoolwork with me. Daddy tells me, 'good job!' And your face just looks like that (pointing to my face), and you don't say anything ... or you fuss at me."

It was like a knife to my heart. Who is this person I have become?

Every day, things happen that remind me of my limitations, but this week they just spoke more loudly than usual. I got a text from my sister, Wendi, who was skiing in Colorado, that it was -14 degrees there! It reminded me of when they first thought that I might have MS. I got a sudden, strange, definitive thought at that time. I thought, "Well, if it's MS, then I'm going on a ski trip this winter with my siblings." Sounds weird, but I love skiing with my siblings. I had a great trip to Utah with my brother and one sister years ago. My other sister couldn't leave her small children at the time. I wanted to relive that with all of us while I still could. Well, the diagnosis wasn't MS, it was "only POTS." So, I didn't plan the trip or ask my siblings to do this for me.

It hadn't occurred to me yet—until I got that text about the -14 degrees—that I'm not sure that I can ski anymore. Even if I could medicate enough to keep my heart rate down and breathe well enough to do it, even if migraines didn't interfere, even if I could balance myself and wasn't dizzy, temperature regulation is a huge issue. And now I feel hurt and angry. Not at anyone in particular, but I guess at the lack of knowledge and understanding about dysautonomia and POTS. If I had been given a diagnosis of MS, I would have known to go and do as much as I could while I still could. But with POTS, it's all so vague. No one really has a clue.

And I'm left feeling like I missed my only chance.

We all process things in our own way. For me, it was a bit delayed. Perhaps it was denial, or trying to push through, or perhaps it was simply the busy business of life. Either way, it wasn't often that I let the grief fill me. One reason I avoided confronting the pain was that I wanted to be someone who did illness well. I didn't want to let POTS change me. Our culture respects people who handle adversity well—myself included. I suppose I not only wanted to *be* respected, but I wanted to respect myself.

But avoiding my emotions was pretty darn stupid now that I think about it. Who says that if you grieve you aren't handling sickness with grace? Who says that you can't shake your fist at God and still handle disease admirably? God can certainly handle it. So, who cares if there are people who can't?

He can handle our questions, our frustrations and our grief. He just wants us to bring it all to Him.

I had learned to lean on God for strength to get through my days, but I still found myself always looking elsewhere for support and *answers*.

The way that I kept myself afloat throughout those first few years of illness was by always looking to the next thing. Maybe at the next doctor's appointment, there would be a new answer. If Greg could just get that raise, then we could hire someone to clean the house. That would make things so much easier! Maybe if we changed the dose of this medication ... I suppose hope is what it was—hope that the next thing would change our situation.

I was learning to depend on God in many areas. There were a lot of things in life that had taught me to lean on Him, but when you can't trust your own ability to stand up ... well, that's a whole new ballgame. From the moment I tried to stand up in the morning, I was instantly and intensely reminded how desperately I needed Him.

God help me. Get me through this day. He must have heard that from me a million times. Through the desperation, I was keenly aware that He was using this experience to draw me closer to Him. At the very least, I was more aware of my constant need for Him. For a long time, I thought that was the extent of what I had to learn from my health drama.

It seemed that just as I'd start to get slightly comfortable in my new situation, something changed. Although it felt like the rug was always being pulled out from under me, I began to notice something peculiar. With each upsetting thing that happened, I went to God. No, it didn't always happen immediately. However, whenever I did finally come to Him, even if I'd struggled and suffered through a lot on my own first, He always had something to teach me through it.

After a while, when the proverbial crud hit the fan, I started to instinctively look for what it was that I needed to learn from the experience. As the days, months and years went on, God kept showing me that I ultimately shouldn't and couldn't be looking for the next thing to help me. Although it would be helpful, having someone clean my house wasn't going to fix my problems. A new medication might do some good, but ultimately would not bring me the peace I sought.

I was looking to Him for literal strength for the day, but I did not see Him as my solution. He needed to be my solution for everything, and although I would have agreed with that statement, I didn't know how to live it ... until slowly, one by one, the things that I looked to were stripped away.

I had once been such a productive person, and now I had to be very careful to pick and choose what activities I did. At first, when I couldn't schedule too much into my week or be on my feet all day, I hated it. It drove me nuts to lay down or sit to rest when I had things I wanted to do. However, after a while, I was too tired to care. Eventually, I learned to even like the fact that my body had forced me to slow down.

Since I was stuck sitting on my backside a lot, I read the Bible and prayed more. Instead of it being a cursory, quick, "get my prayer time in and move on to more productive things," my time reading and praying became my favorite time. The more I did it, the more I *wanted* to do it, and I found myself happy that I couldn't run nonstop.

It seems that in our society—even in Christian circles—it's permissible to spend the afternoon in prayer, reading and sleeping when you are sick. But if you are able-bodied, you should spend your few minutes with God in the morning because once the day starts, it's time to get to work. Being unable to be on my feet gave me the permission I would not have given myself otherwise to spend a significant amount of time with God.

I had also tried to look to finances for relief, but things were becoming more difficult because of my ever-increasing stack of medical bills. Greg was working overtime to try to pay for it all. We weren't going hungry, but I certainly couldn't look to money to help me. It was another area where God was saying, "I'm the answer. Trust Me with this."

Life had been crazy hectic before POTS, and even though I'd let so much around the house go, we were still committed to homeschooling because we didn't have any other good schooling options. It took every ounce of my energy to keep up with this. Therefore, I had zero energy left for keeping up my relationships with friends. I knew my friends were still there and cared, but it took too much strength to even have a phone conversation. It sounds odd, but just focusing on a conversation can sometimes be so exhausting, and I simply didn't have the capacity for it.

Besides, it was so hard to explain to friends what our lives were really like. I knew families who had adopted, who were learning their new children's needs and helping them adjust. I knew families that had children in therapies for various issues, and I knew moms with medical problems, but I didn't know anyone juggling all three at once. (Oh, and don't forget the minor issue of homeschooling while working part-time too.) When I tried to explain it to people, the responses they gave—although meant to support me—made it clear they had no comprehension of what I was dealing with. I suppose I expected that most people wouldn't understand me. Even *I* didn't understand me.

A friend gave me a short devotional book for moms, thinking that I needed something short and sweet. A couple of my friends loved this book and raved about it. It was very thoughtful of her, and I was excited to try it because I did need something *very* short and sweet.

But when I started to read it, I felt more discouraged than ever. I couldn't identify with anything that was supposed to be an encouragement to busy moms. I was a busy mom too, but my life was nothing like the stories portrayed. I couldn't relate to any of their issues. In fact, their issues seemed so trivial to me that they didn't even show a blip on my radar. It made me feel even more guilt and sadness because these were things that I *should* care about; things that my kids probably wanted me to care about.

But I didn't. I couldn't.

Two words: Survival. Mode.

Having no one that I could relate to, not even in books, made me feel incredibly isolated and alone, and intensified my feelings of failure as a mother. It was apparent that I couldn't look to friends to help me through this—not because they wouldn't have tried to be there, but because for many reasons, it just wasn't feasible.

However, there was one person who understood what I was going through better than anyone: my sweet mom.

All my life she has struggled with unidentified health issues. Once I was diagnosed with POTS, we realized that was the source of all her issues all along as well. So, she was undoubtedly an excellent sounding board and had some good advice. I could now understand and empathize with what she endured when I was a child.

There are so many issues that I don't have to explain to her. When things go on around us that others seem unfazed by, we often give each other a knowing look, because it will be driving both of us crazy. She also just instinctively knows some of the things I am dealing with on a daily basis. She has given me prayers that are written out for times that I am too exhausted and can't think clearly enough to pray, because she knows—without me telling her—that this happens a lot.

On the flip side, my mom and I both often try to keep each other from knowing when things get really bad. It's a weird dynamic where each of us is trying to protect the other from increased stress or taking more on ourselves to help the other. I don't think either of us actually buys into the whole "act like everything is fine" gig, but for some reason, we keep on trying.

So, as helpful as my mom was—and as important as family is to me—when things got bad, I felt as if I couldn't always look to them for the help I needed. I know they *wanted* to be there for me, but it either made me feel worse for putting more stress on them, or it was just too hard to try to put into words what I was going through. The times I needed help the most were often the times I felt least capable of asking for it.

Greg was the one person that I wholly leaned on. He has always been an incredible husband and father, but it takes trials to tell you what someone is *truly* made of.

I can't even begin to list all the additional jobs he has slowly taken over as my health has declined. And the thing is, he does every job like he is so happy to do it for me. If he didn't help with such a great attitude, I could easily feel guilty for all the trouble my illness causes him. But instead, by being willing to jump in and take over whenever I need it, he makes me feel more loved and incredibly blessed.

As it became harder for me to keep up with everyday tasks, he took the lead on many things I would have done before, and he was forced out of his comfort zone. He accepted his new role without complaint, even though he never wanted it or expected it. And as a result, it grew his character. He already had a massive load on his plate, and even still, he made it a point to never let the kids feel neglected.

Oh, and get this: he was never someone who was into working out. That was my thing. But in the last couple of years, he has been working out and has gotten quite buff. You wanna know why?

Just in case.

Just in case I should need more help physically, as some POTS patients do, he wants to be sure he is strong enough to take care of me. I mean, come on, where are the heart emoticons when you need them?!

When some people repeat the vows, "In sickness and in health," they picture running to the store to get chicken soup when their spouse has the flu. They don't picture working overtime to pay the medical bills or taking over many of the household duties that their spouse used to do. They don't picture letting their own hopes and dreams go so they can be around to help as much as possible. They don't picture long-term chronic illness that changes the face of your household, your parenting, your marriage, your finances, and your daily and future plans.

Many men would run, but Greg does the opposite. He draws closer, works harder, and loves more deeply. I am so grateful that

God brought him into my life so many years ago, and I don't know what I would do without him.

Are we looking so picture perfect that you want to gag? Well, don't grab the barf bag just yet.

---∞∞∞---

We soon reached a point when it became obvious that the weight of it all was beginning to take a huge toll on Greg. He had to deal with the stress of raising a family on top of his added responsibilities that were taken over to compensate for me. This, coupled with the financial strain and working overtime, were beginning to create significant wear and tear. He became more snappy, moody, on edge, and less tolerant of the kids' shenanigans.

Additionally, Greg was very overprotective of me, and in an effort to keep things quiet and still, he was way too fast to fuss at the kids for just being kids. They would get upset when he would snap at them, and, in turn, this would make me upset— giving me a shot of adrenaline that would zap any energy I had remaining—and the tension in our already highly stressed home rose to new heights.

Of course, to top it all off, children tend to model the behaviors they see. Greg was short on patience due to stress, and I was irritable and snappy due to not feeling well. It was heartbreaking to begin to see them modeling our behaviors.

This was *not* the way we intended to parent!

Although at times I'd get very upset with Greg over his impatience and short fuse with the kids; when I was calm and could think clearly, I honestly felt for him. I couldn't imagine the pressure that weighed on him. I, for one, was very happy that I was the one with POTS and not him. I couldn't imagine being in his shoes, watching the one you love suffer and completely exhausting yourself to do everything you can to help—knowing that it will never be enough to fix the situation.

Emotionally, I could tell that it took a huge toll on him when I had extra bad days. He would seem discouraged and become even more on edge with the kids. So, I started to try to hide it from him. Unfortunately, hiding just ended up making me feel more isolated and alone. Now, I legitimately felt like I had no one to turn to ... except God. *Okay, God. Now it really is just You and me.*

Strangely, even though I felt lonely, I also felt peaceful. I knew what God was getting at here, and I was actually paying attention for once! I committed myself to learning the lesson that He was trying to teach me: that He was sufficient to meet all my needs. Talking to only Him about my troubles proved to be enough.

One week, while we were at church, the teacher asked, "What is that one thing that makes you feel self-sufficient; the one thing that makes you feel not 100% dependent on God?" I knew my answer. It was Greg. Although it seems strange to answer a question about self-sufficiency with the name of another person, he was the one thing that made me feel as if I was not 100% dependent on God. I had become increasingly dependent on *him* since my health started to decline.

Now, before you get your panties in a wad, let me explain. I am not saying that God did not want me to have a good relationship with my husband or family or friends. That is not it at all. God made us for relationships and community. In fact, I believe one benefit of our trials is that it makes us more interdependent.

Besides, God is the One who brought Greg and I together, and there is no doubt He wants us to be there for each other.

However, I believe He did want me to experience a temporary period of having no one to turn to but Him. He wanted me to be forced to experience that He really and truly is enough. It was hard, but I am so thankful for that experience. I would have flipped my lid in the Detroit airport if I didn't already *know* this truth about Him firsthand. It gives me amazing confidence in the all-sufficiency of God, and in turn, I love Him better.

It also gives me the confidence to trust Him with areas that I still struggle with. I can see many blessings that *I* have gained from my illness ... but my children? I'm not so sure.

If I didn't have health issues, I would have been able to spend so much more time playing with them. I would have spent more time in service activities with them. They would have learned the qualities of compassion, service, patience and love for one another through example. I certainly would have invested more time in teaching them to keep up with duties around the house; would they have had a stronger work ethic if I did? I probably would have had the brain power to help them problem solve through their disagreements; to learn to compromise with each other. Instead, I just shut them down. Maybe they wouldn't fight so much now. I wonder how often they have felt like I didn't care about their problems because, in all honesty, I didn't have the energy in the moment to care.

How many ways would their worlds be better if they were not sucked into the alter-universe of POTS along with me? I don't know.

But I also don't know what God is doing in their lives through this. There is SO much I don't know and I can't see.

Have you read the story of Elisha and his servant in 2 Kings? The servant wakes to find that they are completely surrounded by an army with horses and chariots. Justifiably, the servant panics. I don't know about you, but I would have been peeing my pants and crying in the corner.

What does Elisha do? He basically tells the servant to put on a clean loincloth and stop worrying about it. " ... those who are with us are more than those who are with them." (2 Kings 6:16, NASB)

Um, excuse me? How do you figure?

Elisha knows something his servant doesn't. " ... 'O Lord, I pray, open his eyes that he may see.'" (2 Kings 6:17, NASB)

The servant pulls himself together and peeks through one cracked eyelid. Then both eyes fly wide open in disbelief. The surrounding hills are full of horses and chariots of fire. More *are* on their side.

No matter how many times I read this story, I am always surprised by the ending. If I wrote it, it would read, "And then the army of fire flew down the hillside and obliterated the barbarian soldiers who dared to defy the man of God."

Fortunately, God wrote the story, not me. Fortunately for you and I, He is also the one writing our stories.

God struck the barbarian army with blindness so that Elisha could lead them away from their city to Samaria. *That's when you destroyed them all, right God?*

Wrong.

That's when God restored their sight.

And then had the king feed them a huge feast.

And then He sent them back to their homes.

God's ways are not my ways, and that is a good thing. He sees everything throughout the entire universe, throughout all time. I see as though I'm looking through a keyhole, for one moment: the present.

If I were writing my children's story, it would not include a mother with POTS. But I don't know exactly what God has up His royal sleeve. I know that they do have a better understanding of people with invisible illness. They know that sometimes people are unkind, but they still deserve our grace, because they could be dealing with a whole foreign alter-universe of their own. The kids know that it is not okay to judge people, because they have no idea what it is like to live their lives.

I know that as much as they fight and argue and drive each other and me crazy, when they realize that I am having a particularly hard time, they will rein it in, pull themselves together and work with one another to ease my struggle. I know that I spend more time talking with them because I am forced to be still. POTS lends itself well to cuddles and stories about their day. I know that they see a mom who spends a lot of time in her Bible and in prayer, rather than a mom who is constantly running from one task to the next.

And I know that it is better for me to step back and let the Author of the universe continue to write their story. As hard as it still is at times, I must trust Him with their stories.

After all, He has proven to me that He can be trusted, so I'm choosing to believe that having a mom with POTS will create for them an even more beautiful story than they would have had otherwise.

Each of us, each of our stories, are but one broken piece of glass that when put together form an astounding mosaic that tells the story of God's grace and glory. Even the angels—who get to be in God's presence and see Jesus face-to-face—long to see and hear our stories. They can't comprehend what it is like to be so insignificant, so broken, so unworthy and yet, have the Author of all life *become* one of us. And not just become one of us, but also endure our messy, broken lives *with* us, only to give up His life to save us.

Because of what Jesus did, our broken, seemingly worthless, sometimes horrific stories are astoundingly beautiful. In fact, the more horrific the story, the more beautiful it is. How is this possible? Because it is the ugly stories that have the greatest capacity to shine a light on God's magnificent grace and glory. The angels—the perfect angels—look on and wish they could understand what it is like to be given the gift that we have been given; to have a story as beautifully captivating as ours.

That is some amazingly good news. Being broken is actually something to celebrate. The more jagged and broken, the more beautifully my (and your) little piece of glass reflects His glory.

CHAPTER SIX

Humiliation is a Big Word

"But he said to me, 'My grace is sufficient for
you, for my power is made perfect in weakness.'
Therefore I will boast all the more gladly of my
weaknesses, so that the power of Christ may
rest upon me. For the sake of Christ, then, I
am content with weaknesses, insults, hardships,
persecutions, and calamities. For when I am
weak, then I am strong."
– 2 Corinthians 12:9-10, ESV

Some of us are easily embarrassed. I mean, we all get embarrassed at times, but some of us seem to have a much lower threshold than others. Have you ever thought about the fact that if *we* didn't judge other people, we would have much less reason to be embarrassed?

Think about it.

Adam and Eve had no problem traipsing around Eden stark naked until sin entered the picture. Only then did they realize they were naked. Once they understood, they couldn't find themselves fig leaves and perfectly placed greenery fast enough.

If we didn't make our own judgments all the time; if we didn't have negative thoughts toward others swirling around in our minds, we probably wouldn't realize and fear the same things going on in *other* people's heads. If this thought loop didn't exist, we would have far fewer chances of embarrassment in general.

I always thought the fact that I was easily embarrassed was a testament to shyness. Perhaps it was a testament to something a bit more sinister.

Having a mother with POTS causes my children to be caught in ... umm ... unique situations. My oldest son used to volunteer once a month at our county's food pantry, which is held on our church's property. My dad helps organize the event, so he can easily keep an eye on Aiden while he is there.

One hot August morning, we were running late. We live in just about the smallest town in America. In fact, the word town is quite generous. But on food pantry day, it's like trying to get out of the parking lot after a major league baseball game. The cars form multiple lines early because sometimes they run out of food—and let me tell you, those lines are LONG. The police are present to try to keep the road clear and warn oncoming traffic, which consists of about two vehicles an hour that aren't actually coming for the pantry. When the food is placed in an individual's car, they drive around our old school building and leave from the opposite side. The volunteers drive in from this exit side, and since we were late, cars were already coming around the building.

I wasn't sure what to do because I didn't want to get in the way of traffic that was exiting, so I parked in the grass in front of the building. However, from that vantage point, I couldn't see where the volunteers were working or where my dad was because they were on the opposite corner of the tiny two-room school. It was about 875 degrees, sunny and 100% humidity, so I knew that I only had moments out of my vehicle before serious problems would start. I also knew my dad would never respond to his cell in the midst of all the chaos he was trying to orchestrate. I thought about just sending Aiden out and trusting that he would find my dad because hey, this is our church grounds and we *are* in the smallest town in America. But I'm a little paranoid.

I was also afraid to take Noah and Carrington with me because it would be far too easy for someone to start talking to them and slow us down. Or they could spot the playground and decide a mom passed out on the ground wasn't too high a price to pay for a really great slide.

So, I made a decision. It was the only logical decision I saw as a possibility to keep all four of us safe. I sternly warned Noah and Carrington to stay in their seats and not open or unlock the doors. Our windows are tinted, so unless they were loud (which now that I think about it, was a distinct possibility), it would be hard for anyone to even notice them. The van was a cool 72 degrees, and I had pulled into the shade. I put it in park, put on the parking brake, and left the motor running, but took the key fob with me and locked the door so no one could get in. As wild as those two are, I knew I could trust them not to mess with the ignition. I had left no box unchecked.

Or so I thought.

Aiden and I booked it to the other end of the building. I was aware of the sound of tires on the gravel driveway coming from the road, but didn't think it was much to worry about. Besides, I was setting a new speed record for a woman with POTS in that kind of heat.

I glanced back at the peaceful van just before stepping around the side of the school. My dad was a mere 40 feet away, and we rushed over to him.

"You've got Aiden?"

"Yep. No problem," my dad responded as I turned and ran the 40 feet back to the front of the building.

How long could it have taken us to run 40 feet to my dad, for Dad and me to exchange those few words and for me to run 40 feet back? 10 seconds? 15? Let's be generous and say 20 seconds.

There were a mere 20 seconds I was out of sight. When I came back into view, the vehicle that had been pulling into the driveway had parked by my van. I had slowed my pace because not only could I now see the van, but I had just *run* in 875 degrees! I felt like I had just finished a triathlon; I was completely out of breath and increasingly dizzy. I knew I could make it to the van ... I just couldn't run anymore.

I was a bit nervous, however, because a woman had gotten out of the other vehicle and was eyeing my van very strangely. I was trying to pick up my pace, wishing she would move on to the volunteer work that she came for.

And then I saw it.

A sweet little brown hand waving out the window, giving such a lovely greeting to the woman who was now giving me the evil eye. That was the box I hadn't checked. I had forgotten to put the child safety lock on the back-seat window control.

As I approached the van, the woman positioned herself between me and the driver's door. If I tried to write out the dialogue, it wouldn't be very interesting because it was really more of a monologue. I didn't say a word. I couldn't. I tried at first, but she just got more heated and cut me off. And then I couldn't speak anymore because I was standing in place. In 875 degrees. After running.

I wish I could remember everything she said, because she said a lot, but I think I was doing a pretty great job just to stay conscious through it all. I do distinctly remember her saying that she worked for Child Protective Services. I remember her saying that she was going to report me. And I remember her shaking her finger and saying, "YOU HAVE NO MORE CHANCES!"

After that, I remember laying in the van for a long time with my seat reclined and my legs on the dash, trying to restore some blood flow to my brain and sobbing uncontrollably. *Pull yourself together! Noah and Carrington are terrified.* They kept asking what had happened.

"Why was that lady mad at you? What was she saying? Why are you so upset, Mama? What is wrong?!"

Finally, I was no longer dizzy, and I pulled myself together— only I didn't quite pull myself together. That unreasonable, irrational anger that comes from not enough blood flow to my brain was still present, and I did something that I still regret to this day.

I told the kids what she had threatened to do. That she had threatened to take them away. And I blamed them for rolling down the window. Cue all the tears once again.

For weeks, I was afraid that someone was going to show up at our house from Child Protective Services. For months, the kids were afraid that someone was going to take them away ... and that is on me. Honestly, I don't know if that woman truly worked for CPS or not. It may have just been a threat.

This woman, this complete stranger, made a snap judgement. Normally, I would agree with her that you shouldn't leave kids in a van when its 875 degrees outside. Normally, I would have been highly suspicious if I saw children left in a vehicle as well. But nothing is normal about our family anymore.

She couldn't see what lurked below the surface. She didn't know the invisible dangers that our alter-universe presented on a day that was likely perfectly normal for her. She didn't comprehend that in all actuality, *her way* was what endangered us. She didn't know that I made a careful and calculated choice in order to protect *all* of us.

What would my kids have done if I had become completely incapacitated from the schooling she gave me in the heat? And she had no idea how long we were stuck there, waiting. Waiting for the effects of her education to wear off. Thank God we weren't low on gas, the a/c was strong and the engine held up.

As time went on, I started to become more and more fearful of the ways our alter-universe affected our lives, both physically *and* emotionally. How could I protect not only myself, but my children? Now I realized that in addition to having to protect them from POTS, I also needed to protect them from the judgements of others who couldn't see our invisible reality.

One hot day, I pulled into the garage as usual. I opened the car door, and as I was getting out, I dropped my key down between the seats. I reached down, but couldn't get it. My hand didn't fit, and when I tried to bend over to look further, the motion combined with the heat was making me dizzy. I was right in front of the door to the kitchen. Greg and the kids were home, and the house was unlocked. All I had to do was walk inside and ask Greg to go find the key.

But I kept trying to find it and panicked, because I *needed* to be able to do this! I tried as long as I dared, then eventually gave up before I became too dizzy to get myself inside. I walked in, greeted the kids briefly, and then quickly retreated to my room because I couldn't fight back the tears.

I was perfectly safe. But what if?

What if that had happened while I was parked on the side of the street in town? Or as I was getting into the car after it had already been sitting in the heat at the Walmart parking lot? In that situation, I would only have seconds to spare. What if it happened with the three kids? I wouldn't have been able to find the key in time.

And what if our car broke down on the side of the road? Or what if I forgot to take my medicine before driving into town? Sometimes the vulnerability of it all made me feel like a child. I didn't like going anywhere without Greg, and sometimes became frustrated and hurt when he didn't realize how hard or scary a situation was for me. After all, even though he was a part of my alter-universe, he didn't know firsthand what POTS felt like.

Perhaps this sounds like I was being a big baby and needed to suck it up. That's what I felt most of the time, too, and I beat myself up for not being braver.

But then again, someone had threatened to take my children away because of my vulnerability!

Sometimes I thought I was too brave and shouldn't be trying to do the things I did. That balancing act between keeping your family and yourself safe and not giving in too much to loss was a razor-thin edge to walk. Either side I fell on loaded me with a mountain of guilt and made me feel like a complete failure.

We made extra car keys and put spares in my purse along with lots of medication and a cooling fan. I never went anywhere in the summer without cooling towels and my cooling vest in a cooler, even if it was just to the store. Just. In. Case.

We had a medical alert bracelet made that stated "If impaired move to a cool area. POTS. Pacemaker" and Greg's phone number. It hasn't come off my wrist for several years now. In the notes section of my phone, I have an explanation typed up of what is wrong with me, what I likely need, and who to call. Unfortunately, I never once thought to use it when I was in the Detroit airport. If I had, I'm not sure I could have figured out how to find it.

Even still, I learned ways to manage the illness. One thing I try very hard to avoid is being on my feet for long periods of time without breaks—at least to sit with my feet up. Laying down is ideal, but when I can't do that, sitting with my legs out helps restore blood flow and makes all my symptoms better.

Every morning for years, I have set my alarm 30 minutes early so that I can take my medicine, reset the alarm and sleep again until it kicks in. That way I don't have to greet the day to a heart rate of 160. I found assistive devices to help, like a chair for the shower during the summer when I'm at my worst and a cane that turns into a seat so I have a place to rest on field trips.

I discovered that eating only a little bit of protein for breakfast helped a lot with the awful morning weakness and fast heart rate. I have eaten two eggs for breakfast for years. I'm pretty sick of them, but it helps me function. Most people with POTS feel worse when they eat because blood is diverted to the stomach for digestion. This makes it harder to get blood to the heart and brain, so your heart beats faster to compensate. In turn, you feel weaker—not only from the racing heart, but because you aren't getting adequate perfusion throughout your body. The same thing happens when you work out. Blood is diverted to your muscles, so there is less available to help your heart combat gravity.

It's crazy to think about the enormous challenge my body has with getting enough blood to all its organs because giving blood is something that I used to love to do. Someone said to me once, "Well, you can still give blood—you sit for that! That's something you can still do."

Um, nope.

We are always working to increase my volume so all of my body gets the perfusion it needs. I can't *purposefully* decrease it.

When I mentioned all the issues I was having with eating to Dr. Sica—especially that it seemed I tolerated protein better—he told me that insulin, which is secreted more by the pancreas in response to carbohydrates, dilates blood vessels.

So *that* was the issue. I could handle some heat, some blood being diverted for digestion and some insulin, but put them together, and they created the perfect storm that caused me to drop from a size 12 to a size 4 in one summer.

He also told me that with POTS it's a good idea to have a little extra weight because it helps you have more fluid available for the heart to pump. He wanted me to gain back at least 20 pounds of what I'd lost.

"Try to put it back on when the weather is cooler."

Um, excuse me? Did hell just freeze over? I thought I heard my doctor tell *me* that I needed to *gain* weight. It *must* be time for that psych eval.

At any rate, I used the knowledge I'd gained about what happens when I eat to help me be more independent by not eating when I needed to function. Sounds stupid, and it was. It was completely unsustainable and unhealthy, but the fact remained—if I wanted to make it through the day at work as an intelligent and competent physical therapist, that required not eating.

If I needed to take my kids to the doctor, nothing but water and medication passed my lips till I was safely back inside my house. Then, once Greg got home and could take over, I'd stuff my face and either collapse on the sofa for the evening or give up the ghost and head straight to bed. Fortunately, my doctors eventually worked together to figure out a good medication regime that has helped me be able to eat more like a human being than a bear going into hibernation.

Between the doctors, Greg and I, we did all we could to plan ahead and keep the kids and me as safe as possible. However, there reaches a point where you've done all that you can do, and still, the dangers remain. I was being smart about things, planning ahead, but eventually, I had to accept that the vulnerability existed and try to embrace it as an opportunity to learn greater dependence on God.

However, there was something else that I could do to help us be safer when we went places, but this one was a real struggle for me. Dr. Sica had given me a handicap parking permit after I asked him for suggestions on how to prolong my ability to be outside. When he discovered that I was having trouble even getting safely into stores, and how frequently it was happening, he gave me the paperwork for the permit.

I went to the DMV and got the permit immediately. I had difficulty even getting inside. Even though I appear healthy, I don't think the lady behind the counter questioned whether I really needed it one bit. I was leaning over the counter, gasping for breath and she looked terrified that I would pass out in front of her. I was extremely relieved to have it.

But once I had the permit, I couldn't bring myself to use it. Because again, what if?

What if someone I knew saw me using it? What if strangers were rude or lectured me in the heat like the lady at the food pantry had? That could be more dangerous than trying to get into the store from a further parking spot! What if I saw someone from work—someone who knows me but doesn't know my alter-universe?

I mean, let's face it, thirty-something, healthy-looking woman jumps out of a vehicle parked in a handicapped spot and *runs* into Target ... doesn't look good. Before I had POTS, that would have raised my eyebrows, too. I wouldn't have understood if I saw someone I worked with—who I know is physically capable of taking care of others in a hospital—appearing to abuse the system by using an apparent fraudulent handicap permit.

It made me think again about how I had judged people who didn't jump on board with my ideas for ministry. How many other ways did *I* judge people, do we *all* judge people, that we don't even think twice about; that we think is normal and justified? And in how many ways do our "normal" and "justified" judgements, unbeknownst to us, affect those we look down on?

In this case, my very own past judgements were hurting me, as I mentioned at the beginning of the chapter. How were they hurting me? Because I realized that if I thought these things of other people, then surely there were lots of others thinking the same ... only now they were thinking these thoughts about me. In today's world of social media, it is obvious how much judgement goes on because people don't even try to hide it, and it hurts us all.

I eventually started to use my handicap permit when I was far enough from home that I felt pretty confident I wouldn't see anyone I knew. But again, much like with my pacemaker incident, I was allowing fear of letting other people down—fear of what others thought—keep me from protecting myself and my family.

I had to keep asking myself, why do I care so much? Why do I care what other people think? Why did I put myself in danger, such as when I was stuck on the ground at camp meeting, before I would ask for help or even let on that anything was bothering me? As was often the case, I processed my questions and sorrow through writing.

(Men sing) Humble thyself in the sight of the world

(Women echo) Humble thyself in the sight of the world

Isn't that how that song goes? Oh, wait. It's Humble thyself in the sight of the **Lord**. I keep forgetting that.

Seriously. No joke. I have literally sung the lyrics incorrectly in my head over and over this summer. Enough times that I forgot the true words. And that's not the only song I've screwed up.

When I was a kid, we'd sing this song in church that went, "Cooperation is a big word ..." My new version has been "Humiliation is a big word ..." One of these songs pops into my head without fail in any public POTS situation.

The crazy thing is, I'm very open about my condition. I'll tell anyone about what's going on. I have no problem telling you that even though I can walk just fine, the second I'm in the heat I vasodilate. I become dizzy, short of breath, my legs start to give out, and if it gets really bad, I have stroke-like symptoms and can't speak. I can tell you that it's happened multiple times just trying to get groceries with my kids, and it's scary. I can also tell you that sometimes I'm fine and nothing happens. I never know which it will be, which is why I have a handicap parking sticker.

I can tell you that. But, if I see you across the Target parking lot, I'm gonna either park in another spot and risk becoming presyncopal, or circle the lot till you're out of view. Then when I leave the store, I'll make perfectly certain you aren't making your exit at the same time.

And the whole time I shop, two competing tunes are playing in my head, "Humiliation is a big word ..." and "Humble thyself in the sight of the world."

I can tell you that today, August 27, 2015, is my hardest POTS day yet. And it's not because I feel bad physically. It's because it's my baby's 11th birthday and for the third year in a row, he is spending it at King's Dominion. My husband and kids are at an amusement park today, and I had to tell my precious, almost as tall as I am baby, that I couldn't go with him to celebrate his birthday. I smiled brightly as I waved them off, and then collapsed on the floor in a puddle of tears. I can tell you that I've cried off and on all day. I can tell you that this precarious balancing act between acceptance of loss and fear of giving in too much to loss is agonizing. But, if you had shown up at my house today, I'd have dried my tears in a hurry and put on my bravest face.

I can tell you about the dizziness and presyncopal episodes, but will do my best to fake being fine when

I have issues in your presence. I can explain to the nurse at family camp my "special" needs in the heat, yet cringe with humiliation when I actually have to ask for her help.

It's funny how patients are always embarrassed by needing help, or an assistive device, by soiling themselves, wearing a gown ... whatever it might be. And as healthcare workers, we always tell them that there is no reason to be embarrassed. Well, now I've walked a mile in their ugly hospital gripper socks. And I agree with every one of them that it feels more like a marathon. I'm embarrassed right along with them.

"Humiliation is a big word ..."

And yes. I do realize what the problem is. And it isn't POTS. It's pride. In my life, usually if I make a choice knowing that God is leading, it doesn't really concern me what the rest of the world thinks. I answer to Him. But, with my personality being a caretaker, I cannot delegate. I'd rather do all the work myself than tell others what to do. (Um ... by others, I mean anyone other than my husband and kids. I've got no qualms telling them what to do.) So being put in the position of needing help, needing to be cared for and having to ask for help, is excruciating. But POTS is slowly teaching me the lesson that *in all areas* of my life, not just the ones I choose, what really matters is

His opinion of how I handle myself. If I invested half the energy that I expend thinking about my self-image on humbling myself in the sight of the Lord, my relationship with Him would be so much deeper. And I know from past experience that this is the solution to everything.

Today as I spent the day alone and crying out to God, I felt so low. I actually felt angry that it's a beautiful day and not very hot! I was wondering if I could have survived the amusement park and if I had given in to loss. Sitting on my front porch, in the midst of my sobs, I looked up at the beauty surrounding me. And suddenly, inexplicably, I was at peace.

And for the first time this summer, I remembered the rest of the words.

"And **He** shall lift you up."

He *was* lifting me up. But first, He was humbling me by showing me the pride in my heart; showing me that even though I thought I was only concerned with His opinion of me, I was actually far too concerned by others. And the only reason for me to be concerned with what others thought was because I was too concerned with my own self-image. And the only reason I was concerned with my self-image was because of the pride in my heart—knowing the judgements I had cast on others in the past could also now be returned to me.

So, what about this sticky business of pride and embarrassment? It was becoming apparent that serious changes needed to be made if I was going to continue to be a part of many of my children's activities. Sometimes the only way to get over what others think is to be desensitized by repeatedly having your weaknesses exposed. It is a humiliatingly fantastic way to be humbled.

Slowly but surely, I started to use the parking permit. Why? Because quite frankly, I became more afraid of the heat and danger to my kids if something happened to me than I was of what people thought. This was a great stepping stone, because it started to desensitize me to caring so much what others would think. When I started to let go of my pride and concern for what others thought, it sparked something inside me that I was afraid had died.

And I began to dream again of what could be possible.

Were there things that I'd all but given up that could be possible with the right equipment? Was I actually willing to put my silly pride aside and just do what I needed to do to enjoy life with my family?

CHAPTER SEVEN

Coasters and Condemnation

"They were saying this, testing Him, so that they
might have grounds for accusing Him."
– John 8:6, NASB

Human nature is human nature, and not much has changed in 2,000 years. Just as the teachers of the law and the Pharisees were always looking for ways to accuse Jesus, we are always accusing people in our own minds. Based on minimal information, we often jump to the worst conclusion when we should be giving others the benefit of the doubt. We make our judgements, and we assume that we are right because we are wise in our own eyes.

Even though we don't *really* believe it, we behave as if we think we are wiser than God. Yet the Bible tells us that even God's foolishness is wiser than our most brilliant lightbulb moments.

> " ... the foolishness of God is wiser than men, and the weakness of God is stronger than men."
> – 1 Corinthians 1:25, NASB

Even though outwardly I may not behave as if I think I know more than God, I am aware of the dark, hidden crevasses of my own mind. In these well-protected black recesses of my thoughts, it is easy to be not only my own god, but to serve as god and judge for everyone else. I'm not referring to major issues here. Merely small, passing moments when I should have even less evidence to condemn, yet still manage to cast my judgement.

I knew these small accusations weren't right. It was something that I fought against regularly. I wanted to think the best of people, and genuinely felt terrible about it when I realized I wasn't. However, even though I knew I was not the only one who had these hidden places of the heart, I never thought that such small, fleeting incidents could cause significant harm. The food pantry lady was definitely an eye-opener for me, but she had been very vocal and forceful with her opinion. Surely if people didn't tell us what they were thinking; if they never spoke their judgements aloud, then they couldn't create such an impact.

Or could they?

Aiden is absolutely, insanely obsessed with roller coasters. I mean, the boy can tell you every single tiny detail about every roller coaster in the world. No kidding. That is one of the reasons that missing his 11th birthday at King's Dominion had been especially hard for both of us.

As his 12th birthday approached, Greg and I realized that we were going to be within two hours of his dream park just days after his birthday. He had wanted to go to Cedar Point in northern

Ohio for years, and we never thought it would be possible. We started to think that northern Ohio at the end of August could not possibly be as hot as southern Virginia that same time of year. Maybe, with the right equipment, I could actually do it.

He was expecting to get tickets to King's Dominion again for his birthday. My favorite home movie of all time may be the one of his face when instead he opened tickets for *two* days at Cedar Point. There was, in his words, "no better gift we could have given him in the whole world."

We were all very excited. Aiden couldn't stop showing us videos and telling us all the details of the many coasters there, taking surveys of what types of roller coasters we liked or predicted we were going to like best. We had brought my grandmother's old wheelchair. I didn't like it, but had learned to handle my insecurity. Ultimately, I was willing to do what needed to be done to make this happen for our family.

It required careful planning. We called ahead of time to be sure we could store extra packs for my cooling vest in the freezer at first aid. I counted and recounted medicine and made sure I had all of the additional ones on hand that were necessary for me to tolerate the roller coasters. One extra benefit to the use of a wheelchair was that I didn't have to worry about getting too dizzy to walk after a ride! Aiden could take me on anything that dropped, flipped, twisted, or turned ... just no spinning.

I don't think I've ever seen Aiden so excited. He had planned out the park and what order of rides he thought would be the most efficient based on how crowds tend to travel when they arrive at the park.

We arrived well before the park opened, and I donned my cooling vest, put a cooling towel around my neck and tied one around my head. I awkwardly plopped in the wheelchair and set my eyes straight ahead, determined not to focus on anyone but my family.

We had to go to guest relations first to obtain a disability pass. With this pass, instead of waiting in line, we could present it to the attendant at the entrance to the ride to receive a return time that is equivalent to the current estimated wait time for the ride. Even with the wheelchair, it didn't take long in the lines of loud people—or those awful stations where the staff talk into the loudspeakers—for me to feel disoriented and have a migraine kick in. So, the idea of the pass is great and should be fair to all.

After obtaining the pass, we headed to first aid to drop off my extra cold packs, and then it was off to the races. Greg and Aiden took turns pushing me, and everyone was full of smiles and excitement. After each roller coaster, Aiden had a list of questions for each of us. How did it compare to the other coaster we'd just ridden? Rate it on a scale from zero to 10 based on the drop, the speed, the airtime, and the comfort of the restraints. If we didn't like it, that drew a whole new list of questions. For a kid who spends all his free time designing roller coasters, there was nothing better.

After the first couple of coasters, Carrington was too afraid to ride anymore, so Greg or I would ride something smaller nearby with her while the other rode the coaster with the boys. It was pretty exhausting for both Carrington and me when the two of us were on our own. That sweet little thing did her best to help push me. We had considered renting a scooter, but they were just too expensive. So we did the best we could with the manual wheelchair, taking turns back and forth because Greg and I both needed to ride each and every coaster. How else could the world's future best coaster designer do his research?

The only complication so far was that for some rides, the handicap accessible entrances were not well marked, or if they were marked, the signs were confusing. It took quite a while to find where we needed to go on a couple of them. This made me feel bad that I was slowing everyone down.

The boys and I went to ride a coaster together after we had waited for our designated ride time, but couldn't find the elevator. It was starting to get hot, and Aiden was getting tired from pushing me all over trying to figure out where to go. When we finally found the elevator, I picked up the phone that calls up to the station above. An employee is supposed to pick up and send the elevator down to you. No one answered. After a couple minutes of sitting in the sun, I called again. No answer, but an employee did look at the phone, look over the rail to me sitting below and continued to ignore the phone.

My default reaction was embarrassment, and I felt bad that this was happening to the boys. This dream come true for them should not involve a wheelchair at all, much less the time it consumed. But I really did not want it to take even more time because people weren't doing their jobs.

Finally, someone sent the elevator down. The staff wouldn't allow the boys in the elevator with me, so they headed up the stairs. I found myself very thankful that they were somewhat old enough to do this alone. With Aiden being 12 and Noah 9, it still made me uncomfortable, but I knew unless Noah decided to climb the rail they'd be fine. However, I realized that Carrington and I could not ride anything together that involved an elevator.

The elevator was very slow and would have made a fantastic greenhouse. It was about 20 degrees hotter than it was outside, and it was a huge relief when I finally reached the top. I opened the door and started to wheel myself out. An employee held up his hand for me to stop and pushed the door closed again. I was shocked. I had half expected an apology when I came out for how long they took to send it down in the first place, and now they wouldn't let me out?! I started to open the door again, and he immediately pushed it shut. Now my heart rate was shooting up—not just from the heat, but from adrenaline in response to anger and panic. I needed out! I cracked the door and told him just that.

"I need to get out!" He then let me open the door, but kept his hand up showing me that I wasn't to come forward any further than just outside the elevator door. I was nowhere near the do not cross line they had painted on the floor. What did he think I'd come up there to do?

He kept us sitting there in the sunshine for several more minutes before he allowed us to get on the ride. After all was said and done, it took an extra 20 minutes to get onto that ride than it would have if we had waited in line. Then it took extra time afterward to get back down through the greenhouse.

I was baffled, wondering what that guy's problem had been. I didn't feel very well after all that sitting in the sunshine and my greenhouse ride. But I was determined to keep going.

We rode a couple more rides that didn't involve elevators, and then we came to another roller coaster with an elevator. There was no attendant at the ride entrance to give us a return time, but we could see the line, and it was almost completely empty. Besides— the wait time listed at the entrance said five minutes. Carrington wanted a break from the rides for a minute, so she and Greg were just going to wait for us.

"We can just leave the wheelchair with Daddy," I told the boys. "Let's not bother with the elevator. I can make it up the stairs."

It was quite a few steps up to the exit, which is where you are supposed to go with a disability pass, but I went very slowly. When I finally got to the top I was completely out of breath, so I leaned over the rail with my pass in hand. Two employees walked past us and looked at the pass, but didn't do anything. I was too out of breath to say anything. We kept waiting. Eventually, another employee asked one of the staff that had walked past us if he had taken care of the pass.

"No. I don't know what to do with that thing," he responded.

The man who had asked the question said to me, "Just give me a minute."

A minute later he came back. "Finally," Aiden sighed.

We thought he was going to put us straight on the ride. We had already waited longer than anyone in the regular line. Everyone who was in the station when we reached the top of the stairs was already gone.

"I'll get you on in a few trains." He must have seen the shocked look on my face because he finished with, "It's okay. You can wait right here."

Duh. Did he think we were going to walk back around to the regular entrance? Apparently, that's what we should have done in the first place. Then we would have been treated like regular people, and we'd be done with the ride already.

"I can't keep standing here," I said.

"It won't be long."

I was stunned. It seemed as if they were purposefully making us wait longer. I didn't have the wheelchair; therefore, I did not look like I needed the disability pass at all. The platform that we were on was very small and directly in the sun. I was getting dizzier by the second and started to feel confused. I slid down onto the floor and leaned against the railing.

"Are you okay, Mama?" Aiden and Noah both wanted to know.

"Yeah, I just can't stand anymore."

Aiden started pacing and wringing his hands, "Why are they doing this?!"

"I'll be okay."

But I wasn't. I was still directly in the sunshine and getting worse by the moment. As people exited the ride, the gate would swing open right into my legs because we had no room. People would apologize and ask if I was okay. It was obvious to them that something wasn't right. Why else would I be sitting in that spot where the gate was going to hit me repeatedly?

"Do you need help?" rider after rider asked me.

I'd shake my head no because I didn't know what to do, and I couldn't explain the help I needed anyway. The park guests were far more kind and concerned than the employees.

Aiden stood by the rail, staring that employee down. He finally came over and said, "Okay, you guys can get on."

Aiden reached to try to help me up. I waved them toward the ride, "I'll wait."

"Are you sure, Mama? Are you okay?"

I nodded and waved them on again. They looked like they weren't sure if they should go, but then headed to the ride. I pulled out my phone. I knew I didn't have much time left. I started to text Greg, and I think I typed a couple of words correctly before I forgot how to spell. Then I started sending him random numbers and letters.

Greg understood though. When you have a wife with POTS who is alone with two of your kids in an amusement park on a summer day, and you get a weird message, it means "I've fallen, and I can't get up."

He got to me soon after the boys got off the ride. He pulled me to my feet and draped my arms over his shoulder, supporting most of my weight as we slowly made our way down the long staircase. He helped me into the wheelchair and pushed me into the shade where I could put my legs up on a bench, poured water on my cooling towels and pulled out my fan. I laid back as much as I could in the chair and tried my best to catch my breath.

"Did the ride make you sick?" he asked.

I couldn't answer, but Aiden filled him in on what had happened.

Greg was livid. If it weren't for the fact that he could no longer leave me alone with the kids, I think he would have marched right back up those stairs, gotten all of those employees' names, and let them know what they had just done.

We were stuck there for a long time and eventually let the boys go ride the same coaster again on their own because I didn't want this to waste all their time. I had tried so hard to hold it together—and was still trying to because Carrington was still with us—but I didn't succeed. The tears just started to roll.

I was so frustrated, so embarrassed, so angry, so hurt.

SO vulnerable.

Again, it happened so fast. We planned and did all we could, but it just took one person who thought they knew something about me that they didn't know. All it took was one judgment.

ONE judgment.

I pray that I have never made one judgment that has hurt someone else as severely.

After about 45 minutes of rest, we were able to continue on about the park. I felt awful though, and tried incredibly hard to hide this from the kids. I was not up to riding anything, which greatly concerned Aiden and made things very complicated since we had to split up so much due to Carrington being afraid of the roller coasters. Instead of her getting to ride other rides, she mostly just had to sit and rest with me in the shade.

Toward the end of the day, I was starting to feel a bit better, and we came to the mother of all roller coasters. Aiden had been talking about Millennium Force for about a millennium. Apparently, it has won the Golden Ticket Award several years in a row, which means about as much to me as it does to you. But to Aiden, I think it means that this coaster walks on water.

When Greg and the boys returned from riding, even Greg had the excitement of a little boy on his face. "That was amazing! You will have to do it tomorrow," he said.

"Mom, I know you don't feel well ... but do you think there is any way that you could ride it?" Aiden asked with puppy dog eyes.

"Aiden, Mom just isn't up for that today. We will be back tomorrow," Greg replied.

I was about to agree, but then saw Aiden's shoulders slump ever so slightly before he said, "It's okay Mom. I know you don't feel well."

A righteous rage suddenly rose up inside me. *That jerk who made me collapse on the ground may have hurt me, but he will not hurt my son! Especially not on his birthday!*

"Let's go, Aiden."

"Are you serious?! Are you sure? You don't have to, Mama."

"Let's do it."

Greg gave me a look that said, *This isn't a good idea*, but I was already trying to wheel myself toward the entrance. We got our return time from the attendant, waited it out and then headed toward the station.

But yet again, we had difficulty understanding their handicap signs. Which way did we go? We figured it out without too much delay, but it was awfully awkward—you basically had to go against the traffic of everyone coming off the ride for quite a long distance on narrow walkways. When we arrived just below the station, there was an incredibly long ramp leading up to it. I knew I was spent and didn't think I had any energy to be much help pushing myself up that ramp. Aiden was willing, but he had pushed me a lot that day, and I knew it would be tough.

All of the people coming off the ride were coming down a couple flights of stairs. There was space at the bottom to leave the wheelchair, so I told the boys, "Let's just leave the chair here and walk up the steps."

"I don't know about that Mom," Aiden looked concerned. I could tell that he was thinking about the last ride. "I can push you up the ramp."

"I know, but it will be okay. It's getting cooler now, and it is shaded at the top of these stairs."

Aiden looked like he didn't approve, but wasn't going to argue. We went very slowly up the steps, resting on the landing. When we arrived at the top, once again, I leaned over the rail, gasping for breath. This time we were noticed right away. An attendant at the far end of the station spotted us, but started to motion for us to go back down. Aiden waved the disability pass in the air so she would know why we were there. The woman frowned and motioned again for us to go back down the steps. We couldn't figure out what she meant, and she wasn't bothering to walk the 50 feet it required to speak to us. Then she motioned for us to go back down the steps and up the ramp. That would bring us to the gate right next to her.

Walking up the ramp would have made more sense. I don't know why I didn't think of that in the first place. Probably because you are always supposed to go to the ride exit when you use your disability pass, and I had just seen all the riders exiting down the steps. It didn't matter that the ramp led a different way because my brain was in oxygen deprivation mode, which makes me look at things in a very black and white fashion. You take your pass to the exit, and I had just seen where the exit was, so that was where I went.

"She wants us to go down and use the ramp," Aiden said in frustration.

"That ... is not ... happening," I said between gasps for breath.

Coasters and Condemnation

"I'll get the chair!" Aiden said and flew down the steps. *What was he doing?* He grabbed the chair and headed up the ramp like a flash. I yelled his name, and he stopped right below me and looked up.

"I won't be ... able to ... get to it."

He had a good idea. He was getting the chair to the top of the platform, but if this woman wouldn't let us come in from the top of the steps, how was I supposed to get to the chair if he brought it up the ramp? He turned around, took it back to where it had been, and came back up the steps to meet Noah and me.

We looked back toward the woman and held up our pass again in desperation. Once again, she motioned for us to go back down and up the ramp, only this time with sharper movements and an agitated look on her face.

I leaned over the rail, stared her in the eyes and shook my head "no." This was NOT going to happen again!

She looked exasperated and finally walked over to us. "You are *supposed* to come up the ramp. That is what I was trying to tell you! You are not supposed to come in this way."

"I barely made it up here in the first place, and I cannot make it back down and up that ramp again. We have come to the ride exit like we've been told." My tone wasn't exactly super Christian, but it got the job done.

"Okay. But next time, you *must* come up the ramp!"

I nodded. *Probably won't matter cause I'm not so sure you'll still be working here next time.* It was unfortunate for this woman that I was more coherent than I had been during the previous incident.

When we debriefed about the coaster after getting off, Aiden was shocked that I didn't think it was the best one in the park. I

163

didn't give it all the ratings that he expected. It was a great coaster, but with the way I was feeling, it was too rough with far too much G-force. It made me feel pretty sick. But I wasn't experiencing anything the same way I had been before I ended up stuck on the ground waiting for that last ride.

———⁓∞∞⁓———

Fortunately, we had one more day. The next day I didn't feel nearly as well as when we started the first day. I would have expected this even if there had been no problems—just from the long day with all the movement in the heat—but that long incident with not enough blood flow really took a toll.

We went straight to guest relations that second morning and asked to speak to the manager. "That is actually me!" the guy behind the counter said excitedly, and then told us something about having been newly promoted.

We explained all of our concerns and told the incidents from the day before, their effects on me, and the dangers they posed with children involved. We stated that since it wasn't just one isolated incident, it seemed that some significant training was needed with staffing throughout the park on how to properly handle those with disabilities and their disability pass program.

The entire time we talked, he just nodded and said, "okay," about seven or eight times. Then he explained that the woman at Millennium Force couldn't move from her position if she didn't have any other staff members there.

"There were two other staff on the platform."

"Oh ... okay."

That was it. Never an "I'm sorry." Never a "This should have never happened." Or "It won't happen again." Never "I will address this with my staff."

All we got was a blank stare and "okay."

It felt like he was saying, "And you're telling me this story ... why?"

I was truly dumbfounded. I thought that the manager would be mortified. Even if I stepped outside of myself, my children, my fun family getaway; as a physical therapist, I was mortified. Do we really treat people with disabilities like this in America?! Being my first experience with giving in and using a wheelchair to make an outing like this possible for my family, it was extremely discouraging, to say the least.

And it made me wonder, how far and how deep do our judgments run? We've eased into this tolerant culture in America of truth being relative; "What's right for me may not be what's right for you," and "Let's all accept each other and get along." Yet even though this is proclaimed as the way we should all be, I see less acceptance, more judgment and more intolerance everywhere I go.

There was but one person in the history of the world qualified to judge. Yet, in John 8, when the teachers of the law and the Pharisees tried to trap Jesus by bringing a woman who had been caught in adultery to Him, what did He do? The law said she should be stoned. It was cut and dry what *should* happen. The weapons of choice were readily available, and the people willing to wield them were also plentiful.

However, Jesus bent down and started to write in the dirt. When they continued to question Him, He stood up and said, " ...

'Let him who is without sin among you be the first to throw a stone at her'" (John 8:7, ESV). Then He stooped down and continued to write—presumably the sins of the people in the crowd.

The people who were there, ready to stone her, began to leave, one at a time until the woman was alone with Jesus. He said, "Woman, where are they? Has no one condemned you?" (v. 10)

"No one, Lord," she replied. (v. 11)

Wow. It didn't take her long in the presence of Jesus to realize there was no condemnation coming from Him.

"'Neither do I condemn you; go, and from now on sin no more.'" (v.11 con't)

Jesus could have publicly announced all of the sins of the people in the crowd that day. He could have sincerely embarrassed them all. That would have taught them a lesson! *You think you're so much better than she is; let everyone hear what you've done!* Oh, that would have been a juicy story! But then it probably would have been located in Song of Solomon, just to keep all of the taboo stuff centralized.

However, Jesus has the love and compassion in His heart to spare the judgers from embarrassment.

And His reaction to the woman? He corrected her. He did. He didn't ignore what she had done.

But first.

First, He made sure she was safe and *felt* safe. First, He made her feel cared for and loved. First, He provided what she most needed.

Then.

Then He forgave her before she even asked. "Neither do I condemn you." (v.11 con't)

Only after that. Only after giving her what she needed most—an encounter with Jesus as her Savior and Provider who loves her—only after letting her know He didn't condemn her but forgave all, did He correct her.

And He had every right to correct. He had every right to judge. But even He did not do so until she was first cared for.

So, what in the world are you and I doing? If even Jesus didn't judge or correct until He had shown love and provided for the needs of people, then how can we cast a quick judgment based on a momentary encounter? Or even on an acquaintance when we don't intimately know the hidden struggles of their lives? What do you and I want to be known for at the end of the day? Being right? Being able to discern a faker? Making certain that people pay when we suspect injustice?

Or giving people an encounter with Jesus? And showing them that He is their Savior and Provider? It does take a lot of humbling on our part, but wouldn't we rather be known for being like Him?

It sure beats being known for being like Cristy.

Chapter Eight

When God Dreams Small

"There is only one thing that I dread: not to be
worthy of my sufferings."
— Fyodor Dostoevsky

Have you ever prayed for something—I mean, really prayed for something—without realizing what you were actually praying for? Or perhaps later you could see that you were too self-righteous to understand what the implications of your request were?

As I've already mentioned, one of my passions (that can only be God-given) is a love for and desire to help those who are less fortunate. Especially children. So, it wasn't hard to be moved by the prayer of Bob Pierce, the founder of World Vision and Samaritan's Purse. "Let my heart be broken with the things that break the heart of God." When I first heard it, I immediately made it my prayer mantra.

The problem is, when you pray for something, you've got to let go of any preconceived ideas about how your prayer should be answered. If we already have an answer on how to make our desire happen, then why ask God to do for us what we can do for ourselves? If we have a solution to our problem in the first place, then why are we asking God to fix it for us? And furthermore, why would He do it? He certainly gets no glory from doing what we are humanly capable of, and in the end, we wind up doubting that it actually was Him who did it anyway.

Making our requests in prayer involves asking God to do for us *what we can't do for ourselves*. If we cannot do it ourselves, then that leaves us not knowing how He, in His wisdom, should answer. If I were capable of coming up with solutions that are just as good as God's, then would He even be worthy of my praise?

Perhaps this is why we worship so little in our daily lives. When we take a good look deep inside our hearts and are genuinely honest with ourselves, we don't trust that God sees more about our day-to-day lives than we do. We don't see God for who He actually is—infinitely wiser than we could ever imagine.

It is maddening to me when my daughter continuously acts like she knows more than me, insisting that she knows the best way to do everything. From her limited experience, how could I possibly understand that she is incredibly hot in the van right now and doesn't need her coat as she gets out? The sun is shining! But Mommy has the wisdom that a weather app instills and knows that a cold front is coming within the hour.

I guess God is letting me participate in the fellowship of His sufferings with me.

How often do I whine to Him that I don't need this trial right now? *God, don't you understand that I'm already hot from all the fires I've got going? I'm trying to put some out, not light more!* But He has the wisdom that being the Creator of the universe instills. He knows that I need this trial to develop the perseverance for the front that the devil will be bringing on me soon. And as any parent knows—and my Heavenly Father certainly knows this about me—some of us have to learn the hard way.

In praying the prayer, "Let my heart be broken with the things that break the heart of God," I thought I would be given more empathy, compassion, a greater drive to do more and the strength to persevere. I didn't ever want my usefulness to others to be paralyzed by compassion fatigue. It was easy to ask God to up the ante a little on the things that I already cared about; the things that already broke my heart. It was even easier to pray that He would break others' hearts in the same way. After all, many people were lacking in this area. But He answered my prayer by doing the exact opposite of what I expected.

He broke my heart with the things that break His heart by breaking *me*.

A benchmark for me each year was our annual trip to family camp—not to be confused with the camp meeting that we also attended. This was like a kids' summer camp, except it was a week dedicated to the entire family.

Things had changed slowly over time, so sometimes I didn't even realize how many abilities I was losing.

Until it was time for camp.

Each year I was shocked at how much harder it was to make it up those hills. I went from charging up and down them while carrying children and talking to friends, to going slowly, to going slowly while panting for breath, to needing help for balance at times, to often using our van to drive up and down. As someone who always prided myself on being physically fit, I hated it when anyone was walking near me because I was embarrassed that they would think that I was totally out of shape.

For so many years, even though I was miserable, I tried my best to go to as many activities as I could. To not go would have made me more miserable. However, each year, I ended up going to less and less. Eventually, I hardly attended anything, but what was even more upsetting to me was that I was no longer disappointed by it. It used to make me so sad when I couldn't do something; I couldn't stand to miss doing anything with the kids.

I remember one day that I decided to stay and rest while Greg and the kids went on a hike to a waterfall. It was a tradition of ours to hike to those falls every year. It was the most logical thing for me to stay, as I was exhausted from the week and we had to pack up and go home the next day. We didn't think I would make it very far on the hike anyway.

But instead of resting, I spent the entire time that they were gone crying because I was so upset that I couldn't do it. I wished that I had taken my Kindle and just gone however far I could and then sat to read until they finished their hike and returned. At least I would have been a part of it in some capacity.

However, I eventually reached a point where I was so weak and tired that even thinking about trying was too exhausting. I didn't go to activities or on hikes, and it no longer made me sad. I was just so tired that I no longer had any desire to keep pushing myself to do it. When I realized that just staying in the cabin didn't make me upset, I was even more sad!

It was just another incident that made me wonder who I really was now. I knew I wasn't depressed, so that couldn't explain it. But what happened to the girl who loved being with people and didn't want to miss out on a thing?

One day during lunch at camp with a couple friends, we were talking about Myers-Briggs personality types, and someone brought up mine. The two friends with me stopped and looked at each other confused for a minute. One said to me, "You know, I used to have your personality figured out, but it's strange; it's like its changed. I'm not sure what type you are anymore."

I'm not sure either. There is a lot that I don't know anymore.

Throughout my illness, God had drawn me closer to Him, and I had learned that He was enough to meet my needs. I looked to Him for strength and called out to Him for answers. I asked Him to meet my children's needs because I felt that I was failing them in so many ways. I truly wanted to learn what lessons He had for me, because if I had to go through this, I at least wanted to glean what good I could from it. He was teaching me that blessings hide within heartache.

But what about now?

Now, the grief was hitting me in a whole new way—so I decided it was time to seek Him in a new way. I didn't just need Him to help me endure my illness; I needed Him to teach me *who I was* in the midst of it. I had lost myself entirely. I didn't like who I currently saw in the mirror, and I knew, short of a miracle, who I used to be wasn't a possibility anymore. So, the only other option was that God was making something new. Rather, He was making *someone* new.

> "Assuming that you have heard about him and were
> taught in him, as the truth is in Jesus, to put off your

old self, which belongs to your former manner of life and is corrupt through deceitful desires, and to be renewed in the spirit of your minds, and to put on the new self, created after the likeness of God in true righteousness and holiness."

– Ephesians 4:21-24, ESV

"He has made everything beautiful in its time. Also He has put eternity in their hearts, except that no one can find out the work that God does from beginning to end."

– Ecclesiastes 3:11, NKJV

God had been giving me gentle hints that maybe the old Cristy I was oh-so-attached-to wasn't as bright and shiny as I liked to think. POTS or no POTS, there were things about the old me that needed to go—health issues simply forced a sort of "putting off" of my old self.

The next step appeared to be having my attitude made new. I didn't have a *bad* attitude necessarily, but there must be something more to it. I didn't know exactly what God was doing in my life. I could not fathom how He could possibly make something beautiful out of the alter-universe that I was living in, or of the stranger that I had become. However, based on scripture and my relationship with Him, there were a couple of things that I did know.

He *was* making something new, and He *never* makes mistakes.

·⊂∞⊃·

After Carrington had been home a little over a year, life was crazy but wonderful. I was still struggling with some symptoms, but they were mild, and I was choosing to ignore them for the most part. I had never felt so fulfilled and happy, and I wrote about it on our adoption blog.

> I have discovered that the thing that brings me the most joy in life is to follow what God calls me to do. Nothing compares.
>
> Nothing.
>
> This is when I feel the most alive, fulfilled, joyful, patient, loving ... the list could go on and on. So, imagine my confusion a few days ago when someone who is very close to me said, "At some point, you've got to start living your life."
>
> Huh?
>
> This statement was said after a discussion about how Greg and I want to adopt again someday. Now I KNOW that I often don't look like the picture of joy and fulfillment. I know that, God forbid, you should happen to see me in Walmart with three kids, you would see a redhead racing down the aisles like a mad woman, yelling at her kids to stop touching things. You'd likely see a woman who looks haggard, stressed

and just plain exhausted. I know that even in church, my face shows the stress of keeping my two littlest littles from killing each other (we don't even shoot for quiet; no bodily injuries and we call it a success). I am not naive to this fact. But I'd like to bring up an old, worn-out saying.

You can't judge a book by its cover.

Or more importantly, what you believe is truly living might not be what someone else believes truly living is. Yes, I am exhausted. Yes, I am sometimes stressed (okay, a lot of times). Yes, sometimes I just need to NOT be needed! But, BUT, I am also more fulfilled than ever before. I am more confident than ever before. I have an inner joy that I have never known before because my fulfillment, confidence and joy are not based upon circumstance, or even screaming children. They are based on living the life that God has given me, on pursuing the things that HE places on my heart, and on knowing that I am never doing this of my own strength.

Never.

At a graduation speech last year, the question was asked, "What's the one thing you want out of life?" My immediate answer, "To live in the center of God's will." Because I know there is NO greater joy.

That's all I need to feel like I am really *living my life*.

And for the first time, I feel like the expectations or criticism of others can't touch me. I was just confused by the statement mentioned above, and sorry that this person did not understand what "living my life" means to me. That I'm not waiting for something better (other than heaven of course). I wasn't angry, defensive or hurt. I really only have one person to answer to. And that brings a peace that I cannot explain. I know who I am. More importantly, I know *whose* I am.

And I'm so happy to be living my life.

Looking back, it was easy to see how close I was to God. I still knew who I was, and I was proud of the place I had come to in my faith. I felt like I had achieved a new level of trust in Him when I responded so quickly to the graduation speech question with "to live in the center of God's will." I felt like this answer showed the depth of my commitment, and that I genuinely had my priorities straight. I was ready for missions and a life of service. All He had to do was say the word, and I was ready. I wanted to do anything for Christ.

But I never expected the anything to be chronic illness.

However, hardships make fantastic mirrors. They reveal to us who we truly are—not just because they are capable of revealing our strengths, but because they expose our weaknesses and flaws. They have the ability to bring out the ugliest of our uglies. As much as we try to avoid looking, as much as society tells us to buck up and power on, sometimes we have to pause, look straight in that mirror and take in every wart, pimple and blemish.

God has a way of using the worst parts of our lives to break down our sense of control, self-sufficiency, superiority and pride.

Of course, I would have denied the idea of feeling superior or prideful back then. I couldn't see it when my life was secure; when I was capable of helping others, and I was the one in control. I did realize that I loved being in control, but doesn't everyone? And how do you even change that? And of course, I was proud of being self-sufficient. After all, that is an admirable trait in our society. Shouldn't everyone strive to be self-sufficient, like me?

Now, after having my self-sufficiency ripped out from underneath me, I absolutely understand how hard it is for the ones who need help to receive that help. It really is better to give than to receive. I now know what my patients feel like: the vulnerability, the awkward embarrassment, the humiliation of needing to be cared for.

Since the work that God had allowed me to participate in had brought me so much joy, one of my biggest griefs early on was the loss of the ministries that I cared about. I had envisioned that we would never have an empty nest; we would always have foster children or someone running amok in our home. It pained me that I couldn't do church services for Compassion and that we weren't going to live in Rwanda. In fact, I didn't know how I would even handle a trip to visit Rwanda. I couldn't be in the heat! We had also wanted to adopt again, and I grieved for our family and the child that we were never able to bring into the Maddox clan.

When we adopted Carrington, we were blessed not only with a daughter but with a tight-knit community of families who have adopted from Rwanda. Throughout my time of grieving all my lost dreams, I painfully watched the lives of these families unfold before my eyes. Many of them adopted again, several moved to Rwanda and did incredible work there, some started charities in Rwanda, and many continued to make trips there.

I had big dreams that they all seemed to be living. Big dreams that I had believed were also God's dreams for me.

We always think of God as being big and grandiose, don't we? So, it would make sense that His plans and dreams for us are bigger, grander and sexier than our own. Right? Or are they? What happens when your dreams for your family, your ministry—even yourself—are bigger than God's dreams for you?

It can feel like a slap in the face. Pure and utter rejection. It's demoralizing. I'd even go as far as to say it's dehumanizing. All of a sudden, you're 12 again, and the middle school bully has his eye on you. You can hear the laughter of your peers as he taunts, "So, you thought you were something special? Well, look at you now. You aren't good for anything."

The worst part is that, although you know that the bully's name is Satan, it feels an awful lot like God is the one rejecting you. At the very least, He is not doing anything to help you. He obviously wasn't impressed with your life, and did not care about the things that you wanted to do for Him. You were tossed aside, while the apparently worthier ones rose to the top. Your prior resume of faithfulness didn't seem to be considered. You begin to question your own devotion, character and motives. And you shrink smaller and smaller till you can hardly hear your own voice. Silenced.

It is easy to remain there. Silenced. It is a sad, lonely place. But over time it can become strangely comfortable. Comfortable in the sense that it is easier to stay there than to fight your way out. After all, that bully is bigger and stronger than you are, and when you muster the courage to speak, he screams all the louder.

Incapable, useless, weak, a burden, a bad example, incompetent. There are a lot of adjectives he likes to scream.

SCREAM.

And yet, God whispers.

But the great thing is that He whispers over and over and over again. He does not give up on me—even when I give up on myself. I became convinced that I was of no use to Him any longer. I would do my best for my family; to raise my children to the best of my limited ability and teach them of God's love. But beyond this, I could not see that there was anything else for me. The blinding fog of chronic illness was just too thick to see through it.

I suppose deep inside I recognized that there were some ways in which God could still use me. But they seemed generic and obvious, like telling Buddy the Elf that he was good at changing the batteries in the smoke detectors. I strove to remain faithful in these mundane ministries. I wanted to have a good attitude and not be angry with my situation; I wanted to make the most of it.

But I couldn't shake the feeling that I'd been benched because of an injury.

No, it was more than that. I was no longer on the team because my injury wouldn't heal. Yet I was still doing my best to show up, sit in the bleachers and cheer the team on. Cheering with authenticity was the hardest part. Sometimes when that third basewoman cast all thoughts of protecting self aside and threw her body recklessly to catch an incredible line drive, I would cheer while fighting back the tears.

I could have caught that ball, too.

And there are so many line drives that need to be caught. Why was I benched? What could possibly be the point? There are so many needs in this broken world, and so many people ignoring those needs. You know the cliché: Lord, send me anywhere but Africa. I was dying to go to Africa! To wherever He would send me. To adopt. To foster. To speak for Compassion again.

But I was glued in place. Rendered useless. Why were my desires to serve not valued?

It would take a long time to learn and come to terms with the answer. Ultimately, it wasn't that my desire to serve wasn't valued—it's that my desire to serve the way *I* wanted wasn't valued. He wanted my service, just not with strings attached. He wanted full and total surrender, and for my relationship with Him to be strong enough that I would trust what He chose for me.

Even if I didn't like it.

He gently whispered, "Remember that you wanted to live in the center of *My* will? Did you really mean that?"

One can know logically in their head that God's plan is best, but it sometimes takes years for the heart to catch up. I went back and forth with God for years on this issue. Sometimes you have to endure a lot of pain and take time to process your grief before you are ready to fully embrace the truth.

"Therefore we have been buried with Him through baptism into death, so that as Christ was raised from the dead through the glory of the Father, so we too might walk in newness of life."

— Romans 6:4, NASB

Walk in newness of life.

It certainly did take a lot of strength for me to accept my new life and His plan. But actually *wanting* to live in the center of His will, even when it was a far cry from *my* will, was something about me that needed to change. I needed to fully embrace God's dream for my life, no matter how drastically it conflicted with my own, and no matter how noble or admirable my own dreams were. I needed to stop debating with Him all of the benefits of my plan and recognize my need for Him to choose. There is great rest and peace in finally believing and embracing that His plan is best ... even when it's small.

Because even though God's dreams for us are always bigger and better than our own, sometimes that "bigger and better" is pretty darn small. Sometimes it's not a sell-all-you-have-and-move-to-the-ends-of-the-earth kind of dream. Sometimes it's not a fill-your-home-to overflowing-with-anyone-and-everyone-in-need level of service.

Sometimes it's taking your very body, your very health, and laying it at His feet and saying, "Here it is. It really is all that I truly own in this world. It is the most important thing that I have to accomplish big, important things for You, but it is Yours to take. And if in the taking, it means that I live a small life—one that does not involve big, fantastic, admirable dreams, but that does involve

Your glory being revealed in the broken, barely recognizable remnants of what I still cling to—then I will muster the strength each day to say, 'That is my big dream too, God.'"

> "For I consider that the sufferings of this present time are not worthy to be compared with the glory that is to be revealed in us."
>
> – Romans 8:18, NASB

CHAPTER NINE

Beyond the Breakers

*"Therefore we do not lose heart. Even though our
outward man is perishing, yet the inward man is
being renewed day by day. For our light affliction,
which is but for a moment, is working for us a far
more exceeding and eternal weight of glory, while
we do not look at the things which are seen, but
at the things which are not seen. For the things
which are seen are temporary, but the things
which are not seen are eternal."
– 2 Corinthians 4:16-18, NKJV*

Part of the reason I felt that I lost myself in my illness was because I had found so much of my joy and satisfaction through service. It was invigorating to know the help and life I was bringing to others when God used me to find a child a sponsor through Compassion. Although fostering had been incredibly difficult, it brought me peace knowing the pivotal role we were able to play in our foster son's life. Now it seemed my biggest accomplishment was being able to take a shower without sitting down.

After being home from Rwanda a few months, someone questioned if I fostered, worked for Compassion International and even advocated for adoption to fill some sort of void in my life. *What?!* I was astonished that someone could say something like that. I didn't feel like I had a void that needed to be filled—in fact, I had never felt so full!

I pondered on the statement for a while, and then I wrote this in response. I feel it captures my passion and drive that, for me, truly defined who I was.

> I have heard it said that some think I do what I do (sponsoring, fostering, advocating for adoption) to fill some void in my life. Quite frankly, this hurts. It's not that I care that much what people think of me. It's that I want them to understand that it is the joy of the Lord and His love that makes me want to do what I do. Although these things do bring me **immeasurable** joy, I don't do them to fill a void. I do them because of the joy, fulfillment, and peace that I have found in God. And I can't help but want ... but **long**, to help those He loves as much as He loves me. When I have been so blessed, how could I not want to share it?
>
> And it is addicting!
>
> Perhaps that is why some think I'm filling a void, because I always want to do more. And I suppose I will never be satisfied with what I have done. No. As long

as there are starving children and orphans, I will never be satisfied.

Satisfied? No.

But filled with peace and joy? Yes.

I think being satisfied with the little bits we do can be dangerous. It leads us to give a little here, text the word "Haiti" to give $10 there, perhaps even sponsor a child ... and then pat ourselves on the back and say, "Well, at least I did something," all the while missing some other need that we could be filling.

A while back, I began praying that my heart would be broken by the things that break the heart of God. This is where it has led me. It has brought me so much joy. But I cannot pretend that it has not also brought pain. My thoughts and dreams are often filled with the faces of the children left behind. My heart aches for them. I long to do more. So, perhaps wanting to do more is to fill a void, the void of a child who goes to bed hungry, the void of a child who works full time at the age of five to earn one meal a day, the void of a child with no family to call her own. These are God's children. And my life is so full because of my God. WHY NOT use my fullness to fill their void?

And in the process, yes, I receive joy. Not a filled void, but joy in the Lord, in His ability to use little old me.

"The world is a dangerous place to live, not because of those who are evil, but because of those that don't do anything about it."

– Albert Einstein

Overall, there were two responses to this post. The first? "Preach it," which came with excitement and full agreement with what I was saying. The second; however, was offense and hurt, supposing that I was belittling some of the ways that people give. This response caught me off guard.

When I mentioned patting ourselves on the back for what we have done, I was most certainly speaking to myself as well. I was trying to explain why it may appear that I was looking to fill something missing in my life, when I was simply wanting to do *more* (and enjoying doing all I could). I was explaining why I thought it was important to always have our eyes open to where God could use us next.

I couldn't understand how people could be so self-involved that they couldn't see it my way.

Wasn't it obvious to everyone that there was an overwhelming need that we possibly haven't tried hard enough as a whole to fill?

And then I became sick.

"So frail, so ignorant, so liable to misconception is human nature, that each should be careful in the

estimate he places upon another. We little know the bearing of our acts upon the experience of others."
– Ellen G. White, *The Ministry of Healing*

Suddenly our whole world revolved around me. My appointments, my symptoms, my tests, my medicines, my needs. All hail the sick Cristy! It was all-consuming. And you know what?

I didn't have a lick of energy to care about those sweet children living in poverty. I just didn't. It's not that deep down the love for them wasn't still there. It's not that I was a heartless person who only cared about myself. It's that our world was total chaos, and I didn't have an ounce of strength remaining to focus on anything other than getting my family through the day.

When I saw videos from Compassion or pictures of children in need, it didn't tug at my heart like it used to. My heart had been scraped raw one too many times, and my nerves were damaged. I was numb. I was numb to poverty, numb to the needs of those around me, and sadly, sometimes even numb to my own children's little sorrows.

I was so sick of my own story that I wanted to puke, yet I had no time or energy to tear my eyes away from the pages of my own narrative. Guilt set in early on because I had become so self-focused. But when I realized how indifferent I was to rest of the world, well, that's the one thing that didn't make me feel numb. It broke me. And I felt completely lost; like I was living the life of a stranger.

Yet, somehow, those people I couldn't understand—the ones who listened when I talked about the needs of children in poverty, but who wouldn't lift a finger—somehow, they no longer seemed strange to me. It was so easy to judge them from my previous position of relative calm. It was easy to care about and help others when I was in control of my life; when every bit of mental energy wasn't going into my own problems. But now I understood them. And I understood how wrong I had been to be so frustrated with them.

So many things in life are invisible. We don't see all the details, but still, we judge based on our own lives and how we would respond. The truth is, no two lives are the same.

> "Who are you to judge the servant of another? To his
> own master he stands or falls; and he will stand, for
> the Lord is able to make him stand."
> – Romans 14:4, NASB

As Christians, we are all the Lord's servants, and each of us answers only to Him. That is a huge relief knowing that we don't need to be concerned with pleasing others all the time (especially in the midst of writing a book about the chaos that I call my life), but it is also an important reminder that it is none of our business how others serve the Lord. Their lack of service, as it may *appear* to us, isn't our concern either. That's between them and their Master.

Often, there are factors that remain invisible to us, such as sickness, poverty, or relational conflict. Thankfully, God sees it all, even when the people around us cannot. And not only does He see, but He cares and is intimately familiar with every minute detail. Each life is infinitely valuable to Him and has a unique purpose.

The small life that God has given me has a purpose. I LOVED my mission work. Though I loved it because I loved helping others, it had quickly become what I built my identity upon. My identity was never meant to be found in anything or anyone other than Christ.

If I was truly honest with myself, I was so gung-ho on changing the world that I was becoming too busy doing things *for* Him instead of making time to spend *with* Him. I was beginning to miss the beauty of the One who made this amazing world in the first place.

And ultimately, what He wants from me—more than anything that I could ever do for Him—is just me.

That's CRAZY, right?! He just wants me. He was missing the *relationship* with me. That is why He made us, that is our purpose; to be His friend and to bring Him glory in the process.

Sometimes the biggest mission you and I should have is getting to know God more intimately—it just so happens that the most growth often occurs in hardships. We come to know Him best through our pain. Our pain produces growth, and our growth and His glory go hand in hand.

> "In Him we have obtained an inheritance, having been predestined according to the purpose of him who works all things according to the counsel of his will, so that we who were the first to hope in Christ might be to the praise of his glory."
>
> – Ephesians 1:11-12, ESV

"Beloved, do not be surprised at the fiery trial when it comes upon you to test you, as though something strange were happening to you. But rejoice insofar as you share Christ's sufferings, that you may also rejoice and be glad when his glory is revealed."

– 1 Peter 4:12, ESV

We were chosen for His glory. Suffering reveals His glory. It's really quite simple.

———◆———

While we were in the midst of our last homeschooling year, we decided to take the Disney vacation we had always talked about. We realized that once the kids were in school, it wouldn't be possible. There was no way that I could do it in the heat of the summer or navigate the crowds during typical school breaks. We had decided long before that if we ever actually went to Disney, we would need two weeks there because I couldn't keep going day after day to the parks. We would need plenty of rest days in between.

I had never gotten so into planning a trip. We would be there in early December, so everything would be decorated for Christmas. We had only been to Magic Kingdom for one day before, and Noah and Carrington were too little to even remember. None of us had ever been to any of the other parks, and we were thrilled!

Honestly, I think I was more excited than the kids. But when I looked at all there was to do, I began to feel the panic and anxiety rise. The boys and I are alike in the way that we want to be able to do everything when we go somewhere. I knew I would be disappointed if I couldn't do things, but I didn't want to slow the boys down or keep them from getting to everything.

As we were looking at tickets, we realized that once you purchased a five-day ticket, it was very little extra cost to add additional days. We considered it carefully and decided to get a ten-day pass. That way, if there were days where I could only last a couple of hours, we wouldn't have to worry about it. We could spread the adventure out over several shorter days rather than me having to push and destroy myself trying to make it through a few long ones. I wouldn't have to feel guilty knowing I'd made them miss out on something.

I was beyond excited now! But as I continued to plan and look things over, I realized that it was still going to be incredibly difficult. I talked to Dr. Sica about it at my next appointment and asked if there was anything else we could do to help me make it through long days with more energy. He suggested using a wheelchair, which I was already planning to do. In talking it out, an idea came up that, for some reason, had never occurred to this physical therapist.

A reclining wheelchair would be perfect.

However, I was certain my insurance would never cover it. Much to my surprise and delight, it did! As I thought it through, I realized that this was going to be exactly what we needed. Yes, I would look stupid, but I was prepared to put all of that aside for Disney. This was our family trip of a lifetime. I could lay down while we waited for shows to start, or even while waiting in line! I could find a spot in the shade and rest while Greg and the kids continued on if I needed to.

I was thrilled about the possibilities with this new wheelchair, and was quite excited to see what it would be like the day they delivered it.

Until it arrived.

It was perfect for what I needed; however, I spent the next several days fighting back tears whenever I was around the kids or anyone else, and crying my eyes out when I was alone. It was one of those unexpected griefs that hit me out of nowhere. *This* was not how I envisioned our dream Disney vacation. Greg and I should be walking hand in hand, while all of the kids' faces lit up with excitement at the fireworks exploding in the night sky behind Cinderella's castle. Or we could even be far apart from one another, running in opposite directions, each chasing and yelling at a different kid who is whining that they didn't get to ride Space Mountain for the fifth time. I really didn't care which, as long as it didn't involve a wheelchair.

I knew how blessed I was to have the opportunity to be going at all, much less for *two* weeks. I knew having the wheelchair was a blessing. I knew the fact that I only needed it to go to amusement parks and the zoo was also a huge blessing. I understood that people go through things that are *so* much worse, and that in the grand scheme of things, this meant absolutely nothing.

But no matter how much I told myself those things, it didn't stop the grief.

Eventually, I said to God, "I don't know why this particular issue is hurting me so much. I know it's not that big of a deal. But for some reason, it's really painful for me. Please redeem this somehow. I'll be able to handle it if I know that You will use it for good."

At that moment a verse came to mind.

> "Three times I pleaded with the Lord about this,
> that it should leave me. But he said to me, 'My grace
> is sufficient for you, for my power is made perfect in
> weakness.' Therefore I will boast all the more gladly of
> my weaknesses, so that the power of Christ may rest
> upon me. For the sake of Christ, then, I am content
> with weaknesses, insults, hardships, persecutions, and
> calamities. For when I am weak, then I am strong."
>
> – 2 Corinthians 12:8-10, ESV

Even Paul had a "thorn in the flesh," as he called it. We don't know what it was, but we do know that God didn't take it away, even though he pleaded. And we know that it had a purpose. As I pictured myself at Disney in that new wheelchair, this verse was a great reminder to me. It was a tangible reminder that this was an opportunity to experience Christ's power, to be filled with His strength, not *in spite* of my situation, but *because* of it.

Therefore, even if I didn't feel like it one tiny bit, I was going to give thanks for my "thorn." I knew that if I couldn't give thanks for it, then I would have no chance of being able to delight in my weakness, as Paul did. I also knew each time I sat in that chair I would feel embarrassed; I knew that I would forget that lesson *and* that verse.

So, I put it on the chair—on both sides. For myself and everyone else to see.

If I'm being completely honest, this made the chair feel even more awkward to me. But that was okay. It was the reminder I needed that yes, I was weak. Yes, I felt embarrassed. But there was a purpose that was far more important than those feelings.

And perhaps it gave it a redeeming quality. I know a lot of people read it. They may have thought I was crazy. But hey, I was already reclining and asleep with a cooling vest on that makes it look like I'm packing a bomb, with my children holding battery-operated fans blowing them on me like I was the queen of Egypt, all while in line to watch the Lion King show at Disney ... so it really didn't make that much of a difference.

And I must say, when it comes to disabilities, Disney does it right. "We have a party of five with a chariot." It was the complete opposite experience from what we had at Cedar Point. And as if I didn't already look crazy enough, I found myself bawling during the Lion King show when my kids were pulled up front to be a part of the performance. They were chosen because they were in the front row, and they were in the front row all because of my "chariot." It was our first show on our first day, and it felt like a wink from God. I felt Him saying, "Relax. Enjoy this. I'm redeeming this for your children as well."

And He did. For nearly every show, they had their choice to sit in the front or back—or we could abandon the chair and sit elsewhere. And let's just say, I'm not the only person who enjoyed a few rests reclining while waiting for the late-night fireworks.

I know it sounds silly, but the experience at Disney and that one act of placing scripture on my stupid wheelchair ignited a flame in me that I thought was extinguished. It was the moment that I truly considered that there might be, could be, ministries that God still had for me—ministries that He even designed for me. Not things that I could still do even though I had POTS, but things that I could do *because* I had POTS. Maybe there were things that I could do to help others that wouldn't be possible without POTS. Maybe God was showing me something new.

Just maybe ...

———

When I was little, my family would go to the beach each summer for vacation. I mostly played along the shore before I was old enough to be a strong swimmer. If the ocean was very calm, I would swim, but when it was rough, letting the waves chase my feet on the sand was enough for me. My dad would try to get me to go in. I would refuse. He would tell me that once we got past the breakers, we could ride the large swells up and down. It would be fun.

But I already knew that. I knew that it would be fun *once* we got out there. But it was too scary to try to get past the breakers.

Occasionally, he would just pick me up and take me—kicking and screaming and begging my mom for help—into the crashing waves. My mom would be yelling at my dad and following after us. Between the rise and fall of the terrifying whitecaps, I could see my sister having fun far out in the blue. Sometimes there would be an uncle or aunt out there, too. Eventually, I would give in and simply cling to my dad for dear life. I was petrified. I knew all too well the horrifying feeling of being drug under, of fighting to get to the surface even while being unsure which direction the surface was. It was always such a relief to reach the family we were struggling toward.

Of course, once we got out beyond the breakers, it was fun riding the swells. I was happy to be with my family and not miss out on the excitement. But, I could never fully enjoy it ... because I knew I had to return through the crashing waves.

As I got a little older and became a stronger swimmer, I learned to love those waves. I logged many hours in the ocean, and sure enough, those whitecaps were suddenly not as scary to me as they once were. In fact, we complained when the waves weren't big enough and thought it was boring when the water wasn't rough. Big waves were fun because they were challenging. Trying to catch them to get a long ride took perfect timing. Sometimes we would work at it for a long time, getting water up our nose, seaweed around our legs and sand in our suits. And sometimes the waves would catch us, and we'd get tumbled and flipped and smacked into the sand.

But occasionally, I'd get that perfect ride that carried me all the way till my board got stuck on the shore. The ride was worth the water-plugged nose, seaweed and sandy suit.

Some of those waves could be intimidating. Even with experience, an extra big one could tempt me to dive through or under it. That way I was sure to avoid being smacked into the sand. But if I did that, I also had no chance of an awesome ride.

Like you, life has brought me many rough seas. Most of the time, all I want to do is stay on the shore. It is safe there; familiar, even. After all, I can still have fun right there, in the sand. I look at the crashing waves and think that it is just so hard—too hard trying to get past the breakers. I have had breakers of infertility, special parenting difficulties, and chronic illness. You have your own breakers. Divorce, lost dreams, regret, abuse, broken careers, shame, death. It often seems that these breakers will break *us*. That they will take us down and we will never come up for air again.

When we get that low—so fatigued, so afraid, so OVER-IT—that we don't even want to fight the breakers, well, that's when our Dad comes along.

He is an expert at showing us that, although intimidating, at times even painful, breakers can give us some of life's most wild rides. But unlike my childhood self, He won't pick me up kicking and screaming. I have to agree to let Him carry me. He won't force me. And just because I get past the breakers doesn't mean that I won't have to pass through the same waters again ... and again.

But here's the deal: when I pass through those waters again, I am more experienced. I've been through this before. Now, the choice is entirely mine whether I use that experience to help me or to hinder me. I can remember the fear, the anxiety, the height of the angry foam towering over me. I can remember and fixate on how awful it felt to be pounded into the sand and gasp for air. Or, I can remember the lessons learned the first time around and how I got through it. I can recognize the growth that has taken place in me as a result of enduring the surf, and, hard as it may be, attempt to embrace the breakers as another opportunity to learn the valuable lessons that God wants to teach.

Because He knows that as long as we are on this earth, the waves will not stop coming. But that is precisely why He wants us to learn not to merely get past the breakers, but to ride them with confidence.

He wants me to continue to praise Him and enjoy the ride because I trust that even if my face meets the sand, my Lifeguard will be there. If I can do that, then instead of spending my emotional energy raging against the waves, I will be able to spend it listening to what He is saying. Because whether I am listening or not, He *is* speaking, and I don't want to miss it.

Those who have been blessed—yes, I said blessed—with many breakers gain more experience with them. With more experience comes not only greater stamina to endure them, but the ability to thrive and learn new skills *because* of them. My battles with literal breakers taught me that it's a lot more fun to catch the wave instead of trying to avoid it by diving underneath.

Even at the risk of being beaten into the sand.

My battles with real-life breakers have taught me more lessons than all my college and university education combined. Sometimes, I think that the best things in life may be hidden in those whitecaps. They are so fantastically disguised as towering, terrifying waves that want to take me down and tumble me till I don't know which way is up. It takes a perceptive eye and vulnerably open heart to God to recognize that they may turn out to be some of our greatest blessings.

But only if we let them.

People often say that you shouldn't let illness or the bad things in life change who you are. I say, if you don't let them change who you are, then you have suffered in vain! You have wasted perfectly good pain.

The truth is, the hard, ugly things of life change us more than the easy, pretty things. The question then becomes, will you fight it and allow it to change you for the worse, or will you work with your pain and let it shape you for the better? Sometimes our worst experiences are merely preparations for our best. Just like with oysters and pearls, it takes some grinding against the sand to make something beautiful in your life.

He was making me new ... but was He also preparing me for something new?

One thing was certain. I had learned that all-important lesson: don't fight the One who is carrying you.

Cling to Him for dear life.

———∞∞———

The more I clung to Him, the more I naturally focused on Him. When I was focused on Him, my focus couldn't be on comparing myself to other people. We all do the comparing game. I really don't know why, because all it ever does is make us feel bad about ourselves.

I know I am not the only person who has gotten off of Facebook thinking, *so many moms are doing xy and z. Should I be doing that?* And then it snowballs with thoughts of all the things that I used to do but can't manage anymore. All the things that I have meant to start doing but forgot. All the activities that I see other people doing that I want to be doing with my kids. *Wow, her house is so clean and pretty. This place is a mess. How am I ever going to get this cleaned up?* And it continues to spiral from there.

I compare myself to other moms, to other families, and what drives me the craziest; to what I had imagined our family would look like before I had POTS.

When I am clinging to and focused on God, none of that happens. When I am focused on Him, I feel His pleasure and reassurance that I don't have to be like all the other families. Not only that, but He didn't make us to be like all the other families.

I am not doing tons of activities with my children outdoors. I don't keep neat chore charts with exciting reward systems. I don't have everything organized and ready for my kids when it is time to go places, we often forget things and we are usually late. I am not the mom who volunteers and helps out at all their school and athletic events. I don't cook great homemade meals like my mom did. They don't enter the house to the aroma of delicious baked goods. We are not the hangout house for all their friends. We do not have people over for dinner or throw parties. These are all the things that I see other families doing, and furthermore, that is what I thought we would do. That is who I thought we would be.

And we are not.

Do you know what we are? We are a hot mess. A disorganized, haphazard chore-having, throwing a frozen pizza in the oven, yelling and occasionally even screaming when we can't get everyone out the door on time, hot mess. If you came here looking for truth, that's the God's honest truth of the matter.

We have multiple ADHD individuals in the family, and I'm not only talking children. It seems POTS has made me more scattered than Carrington's school supplies when we are about to miss the bus. We have issues. And I'm not simply saying that to be cute. I mean serious, ongoing, drama-inducing issues.

But you know what else we are? We are what God has called us to be. No, we are seriously not perfected. He still has a LOT of work on His hands. But we are right where He wants us. A hot mess, with our drama and weaknesses fully exposed. We have to repent and apologize to each other regularly for letting our weaknesses get the better of us. But we are where He wants us because we are all aware of how weak we are. We know how broken we are and how desperately we need His forgiveness and grace. We know how dependent we are on Him.

Our life is not Pinterest-perfect. Our life calls us to be more dependent on God than most other people I know. And that is something that we are learning to embrace.

The crazy thing is that God reveals another weakness to me at times when I am doing better, such as during cooler weather. It is then that I find myself drifting further from God and not even realizing it. When I'm better, I'm busier, and I don't feel my need of Him as keenly. So, slowly but surely—never intentionally—God gets pushed to the side.

I mentioned this phenomenon to my pastor after a period of doing well physically. "Why can't I just be better and still ..." I struggled for the words.

" ... be better?" she finished.

"Yes! I want to be better *and* be better! Why do I have to be sick to stay close to God?"

That last question popped out spontaneously, but it has stuck with me. It's something that is unique to me.

But also, it's not.

Not everyone would need to be physically glued down on their butt to make them invest in God like they need to. But most people do have something that gets in the way—a hidden weakness that is uniquely their own—that if exposed magnetizes us to our Creator. It reveals what we should have seen all along; that we are completely dependent on Him.

We could each ask our own question.

Why do I have to struggle with my finances to stay close to God? Why do I have to feel lonely to stay close to God? Why does it take anxiety and worry to drive me to Him? Why do I forget about God until the painful memories of my childhood surface? It is often displayed in our biggest challenge, greatest fear or most heartbreaking sorrow.

Why do parents make their children go to school, study, learn to do chores or organize their belongings? Those things are hard for kids. They would much prefer to be swinging outside or picking their noses. But we as parents have the vision to see what the future holds. We understand that sadly, childhood won't last forever. We love them enough to do the hard work of making them learn to do all those difficult and boring things, because even though we screw it up more times than we can count, we are good parents who want what's best for our kids. We love them enough *not* to give them what they want.

And God is a good, good Father. He knows what we will face in the future and what we need to prepare us for it. He also has the vision to see what we forget. That thankfully, this world won't last forever. He loves us enough to do whatever it takes, and to use whatever circumstances present themselves to prepare us for what is coming; for what ultimately matters. He loves me enough *not* to give me what I want.

> "'For I know the plans I have for you,'" declares the Lord, "'plans for welfare and not for evil, to give you a future and a hope.'"
>
> – Jeremiah 29:11, ESV

Before I got sick, I had no problem exercising every day. I was always extremely dedicated to my workouts. What I *did* have a problem with was daily time with God. I tried, but it ended up being sporadic even though I knew it should be my top priority. There was even a verse that God would bring to my mind to clue me into how messed up my priorities were.

> "For while bodily training is of some value, godliness is of value in every way, as it holds promise for the present life and also for the life to come."
> – 1 Timothy 4:8, ESV

That verse had a convicting power before I was sick. After I became sick, it was an encouragement. To me, it meant: health is only good for some things, but what I was gaining through lack of health—a deeper relationship with God—was good for everything, both now and throughout eternity.

Wouldn't it be great if life could be perfect *and* we still stayed close to God? It would be ... but it *will* be, because that is called heaven and that is not now. It isn't possible now because we aren't perfect now. We are sinful people, full of selfish and often downright evil desires. Therefore, on this side of heaven, if we want to stay close to God, unfortunately it takes what this broken world has to offer. Sickness, financial struggles, loneliness, anxiety, pain, and death.

And from God's all-knowing, eternal perspective, our happiness, safety and comfort in this temporary life are not the top priorities. If our relationship with God is the most important thing in this world because it lasts for eternity, and if it takes all the awful pain of this world to drive us to Him, then good times, good feelings and a comfortable life are *not* what we need. They are not what is best for us. It is possible that our worst experiences, our greatest heartaches are some of God's greatest gifts.

Our biggest problem in this world may not be our problem at all. It may be our expectations. Jesus told us in John 16:33, "'I have said these things to you, that in me you may have peace. In this world you will have tribulation. But take heart; I have overcome the world.'"

So why do we expect to have a lovely, peaceful, safe life? Why are we so surprised when we have trouble? Jesus said we would. We don't have to be happy about our trouble, and we can even grieve deeply for it.

But we should *expect it.*

Expectations can change everything about our attitude. They can change the way we react to everyone and every circumstance. Jesus even said He was telling us this so we may have peace.

Peace! Is that even possible in the midst of chaos?

When you expect the chaos; when you recognize that God has a purpose in it; when you don't get upset about what you think you deserve to have, then yes, peace is absolutely possible— in Christ.

And sometimes, it's even possible to go beyond peace to what Paul found.

> "Not only that, but we rejoice in our sufferings, knowing that suffering produces endurance, and endurance produces character, and character produces hope, and hope does not put us to shame, because

God's love has been poured into our hearts through
the Holy Spirit who has been given to us."

– Romans 5:3-5, ESV

You are not able to control all the things that happen to you in life, nor should you. You are not responsible for all of that. However, you are able to control your responses. And controlling your responses comes a whole lot easier if you begin with the right expectations.

Expect pain. Expect difficulty. Expect heartache. Don't be an Eeyore about it. But know that the bad stuff is normal. It is supposed to happen. It is, even at times, in light of eternity, good.

One day we will literally be singing God's praises for all eternity, in part because of all those "bad" things that happened to us. There may even be additional friends with us as a result of what we endured.

And I would venture a guess that when that time comes, we wouldn't trade those distant heartaches for all the safety, happiness and comfort that this expired world had to offer.

CHAPTER TEN

Better When Broken

*"You have to thank God for the seemingly good
and the seemingly bad because really, you don't
know the difference."*
– Jennie Allen, Anything

This has quickly become one of my favorite quotes. Why? Because much like Elisha's servant in 2 Kings 6, we can't see the big picture. Oftentimes what we think is bad is actually good, and what we think is good is actually bad: such as my first day of college.

I was thrilled to be registered for a class that was notoriously hard to get into, and I was excited to take it. But in the first class, I was told that I wasn't registered for it at all. As if it wasn't embarrassing enough to be kicked out of my first class, I then found out that the only remaining class was the one I least wanted to take.

However, the only remaining seat in that class happened to be two desks away from the man I've now been married to for 20 years. What started out as a pretty awful start to my first day of college has literally changed my entire life in the most amazing way.

Children are the same way. They think they know and understand everything, and you and I both know the drama and humor this sometimes creates. I will never forget driving along in our minivan one day with my mom and the three kids when they were really little. I randomly mentioned to Mom that Noah had diarrhea. Instantly, Carrington began yelling from the backseat, "I want diarrhea too!" As we burst into hysterics, her yelling became frantic screams trying to articulate her desperate need to have diarrhea.

Noah had it. She didn't. Simple.

It was so unfair.

What a horrid mother I was.

When Aiden was nine, he said very seriously, "I figure I know about half of everything there is to know in the world by now." Without missing a beat, Greg replied equally as seriously, "Well, you are halfway to 18, so that makes perfect sense."

Don't you just wish that somehow they could understand how much they *don't* understand? If that were the case, rather than being angry that you won't give them diarrhea or getting their feelings hurt when you laugh at them having half the world's knowledge, they would be able to say, "I don't get it Mama, but I'll trust you."

As I was in the midst of working on this chapter, I was putting the kids to bed one night, and Noah said something that made me think long and hard.

"If you could *not* have POTS, Mama, would you do it? I mean, what would you pick?" In typical Noah dramatics, he threw one arm to one side as he said, "Would you choose POTS," his other arm flew to the opposite side, "or would you choose freedom?"

I sat and stared at him in disbelief for a moment. *Freedom, huh? Interesting choice of words there, buddy.* Oddly enough (or not odd at all if you think about it), this was the exact subject I had been pondering with the Holy Spirit as I thought about Paul's thorn in the flesh. I thought seriously about how he also gave up his literal freedoms willingly, and in turn, God used it to draw people in and glorify Himself.

When I think of something that we view as a detriment eventually turning out to be good, Paul is one of the first examples I think of. Paul was no small missionary. He was spreading the gospel of Jesus like wildfire. He was bringing untold numbers to Christ. He was warned by the Holy Spirit that prison and hardships awaited him and even so, the Spirit still compelled him to go to Jerusalem. A prophet even prophesied that the Jews in Jerusalem would imprison him, and his friends begged him not to go.

Paul had every reason in the book to back out of going. It wasn't a good idea to risk his ministry. What about his obligation to all those he had already brought to Christ? He still needed to be available to encourage them. What about all the people he could still bring to Christ? It made zero human sense to go. It was a bad idea, plain and simple.

But Paul went to Jerusalem anyway, because as he had said, "But I do not account my life of any value nor as precious to myself, if only I may finish my course and the ministry that I received from the Lord Jesus, to testify to the gospel of the grace of God" (Acts 20:24, ESV).

And the worst happened. Or maybe it was the best. How do we really know?

Paul was imprisoned. For years. The greatest missionary there ever was, and he could no longer go on mission trips. How could God let that happen?

During Paul's missionary journeys, he was usually far from the people he cared about. In fact, he wrote to many of the people he had shared the gospel with about how much it saddened him that he had not been able to get back to visit them. He could only be in one place at one time. He didn't have Facebook or blogs to communicate with his following or to get the word out to more people.

However, during his imprisonment, Paul was able to share the gospel with some pretty high-ranking dudes. Felix, Festus, King Agrippa. He was moved from place to place, sometimes with an entourage of 200 soldiers. He caused quite an uproar, which created much interest in him. Soldiers rotated positions, so he always had new people to share with. These soldiers then moved on to new places themselves, and the gospel continued to spread. It's was Paul's form of social media. He didn't have a Facebook post button, but he could tell all the people around him about Jesus and watch the message go viral as those people traveled on. Paul's platform and audience *grew* from being imprisoned.

Who would have thought? Certainly not you or me.

But God did.

As I began to accept my POTS imprisonment, learning that it wasn't *all* bad, I began to wonder if even more good could come from it. Could something that looked depressing from the outside, like a prison, actually be good in a way that I hadn't envisioned yet? It seemed impossible.

But God.

When we were in the middle of our last year of homeschooling, I began to think more and more about what my life would look like once the kids were in traditional school. The thought of them starting school made me sad, happy, nostalgic, excited and nervous all at the same time. There were so many emotions. It also brought up some old grief that I thought I had moved past. Before POTS, I always thought that once we finished homeschooling and the kids were a little older, I would work more to help pay for their school. I would get back into volunteering with Compassion International. And let me tell you, my house would *finally* get organized.

It was very clear that I couldn't work more. Yes, I could get through extra days from time to time, but not without it being detrimental to my health, and therefore damaging to my mothering and the health of our family. I could organize tiny bits at a time, but all my plans for action were significantly limited. Maybe I could do something with Compassion, but it would mostly consist of posting online.

I began to pray earnestly about what God wanted for my days when the kids were in school. I didn't know how much time I would have available, but I knew I would have more than I did while homeschooling. However, at first, my prayers did not have an expectant, God's-got-something-for-me, anticipation. They were a sad, what-can-You-do-to-help-me-not-feel-so-bad-about-this, type of prayer.

Yet, something strange began to change in my heart after that simple act of putting scripture on my wheelchair. I could feel God speaking to me and saying, "I've still got something for you."

I couldn't imagine what that something could be, and frankly, I didn't really believe it.

One day I looked up at a chalkboard that is on my wall. On it, there was a verse written that has been up for a long time. I've heard it my whole life, and even memorized it as a child. However, I couldn't believe that I had never noticed something about it before.

> "For we are His workmanship, created in Christ Jesus for good works, which God prepared beforehand so that we would walk in them."
>
> – Ephesians 2:10, NASB

Prepared beforehand.

Why had I never paid attention to those two words in light of my current circumstances? God knew that I was going to get POTS. He knew every single trial that I would face. Even so, He had prepared good works *beforehand* for me. This meant that even though all my plans had been derailed, God's hadn't.

He did have something for me. I simply had no idea what it could possibly be.

Several months later, after I had been praying a lot about what God had prepared for me, I started to feel like He wanted me to write. This didn't totally surprise me—I had done a little blogging in the past, and I liked to write. It was something that I could do from the comfort of a seated position on my own couch. It was doable.

At least, *my idea* of writing was doable. I thought He was asking me to blog. Yet even that, although possible, I didn't like the idea of doing. But I went ahead and wrote my first post. Here is an excerpt from it.

> Our church has focused lately on what specifically God is calling us to do. It is one of those subjects that kinda steps on my tingling potsie toes because I have felt so paralyzed by my health in this area. I can't do the big things that **I** wanted to do for God. And the small stuff... being a good wife and mother, doing your very best at your job, loving your neighbor, blah blah blah. That stuff is ... well, isn't that a given? Shouldn't everyone do that? Christian or not?

> Although I know that stuff is extremely important and has huge value, I've struggled. I wanted to do so much more. I have had to learn to be satisfied with where I am. To see that this "small" life can be huge all on its own. And let me tell you, that small stuff is not so small when you are sick.

> As my church has focused on what God is calling us to do, I keep thinking about how limited my options are. But writing keeps coming to mind over and over again.

Before I got sick, I was up for anything He asked. But sometimes the anything He gives us comes in smaller, less sparkly packages. And I know that writing is a small thing. So why does it feel so huge? I suppose this is a perfect example of the difference in life before and after POTS.

I don't know exactly where this blog thingy is going, how often or for how long I will write. I just know that I feel God is telling me to write and so I want to take the first step of obedience. There are many subjects that God has given me a passion for. I know I want to raise awareness for this illness that has transformed my life. I know I want to show an uncensored view of how rough it is. But I also want to show some of the beauty that God has created from it. Beauty that wouldn't exist if POTS did not also exist in my life.

I had my first post written, so I should have been all set. But I could never bring myself to push the post button. I didn't know what was holding me back. Something didn't feel right, and I honestly didn't believe that I was making excuses to get out of following through. I fully believed that God wanted me to write, so why did something stop me every time I tried to post it? Although a fear of commitment and worry for the time it would require had concerned me at first, that wasn't what was scaring me at this point. I was willing to do whatever I needed to, because more than anything else, I wanted to bring glory to my amazing God.

After all, that was the purpose of my life before POTS, and that is one of the few things that POTS cannot touch.

I was stumped. I didn't have any idea the lengths that God was asking me to go to in order to write for Him. He got me to commit to writing, but I didn't have the full picture yet.

Sometimes God is sneaky like that.

—————∞∞∞—————

I never planned to write a book. It wasn't on my bucket list. It was never something I aspired to do. True, I did have a teacher in college who tried to convince me to be a writer, but I had laughed in her face.

Respectfully.

I had *respectfully* laughed in her face.

Because who would want to be a writer anyway? That involves sitting, and sitting behind a computer no less. That was definitely not something that I would ever do.

But have you ever considered the possibility that not only can God use your pain to draw you to Him and teach you, but that He can also turn your greatest trial into your greatest adventure? Think about it. It's just the kind of insane thing that our ridiculously lavish God would do.

And this? This crazy, absurd miracle that you hold in your hand is a great adventure that God took me on. I couldn't push the post button on my blog because blogging wasn't what He was asking of me. If God had been sitting on my couch when He started to tell me that He wanted me to write a book, I'm afraid that I may have laughed in His face as well. Possibly even spewing coffee out of my nose onto His royal white robe. But I'm pretty sure after that, He would have been cracking up right along with me.

It was an absolutely ludicrous notion to me.

So, God had to tell me again.

And again.

And again.

And again.

He told me through prayer, through the Bible and through book after book that I picked up. I asked Him so many questions—very specific questions—almost challenging Him. *Okay God, if you really want me to do this then try and answer this* ... And much to my dismay, the next book I would pick up, sermon I would hear or scripture I read would have a very thorough, specific answer to my question. Over and over and over again.

It almost became comical. I'd literally laugh out loud sometimes because it was so ridiculous that He had answered, so clearly, yet again. And still, I was telling Him no.

There was no way I was going to do this!

After months, I finally worked up the courage to tell Greg about what was going on. He was way too annoyingly enthusiastic and immediately took God's side ... so much for the two shall become one. He encouraged me to talk to a friend who is a writer, Alison, about it.

"No way," I told him. There was absolutely no way I was ready for that. "Besides, I'm only 99% convinced. I've told God that I want someone to tell me I should write a book or ask me to write for a book. That's what I need to be totally convinced."

"You should write a book," Greg said sarcastically.

"You don't count! It needs to be someone who has no idea about any of this. Which is basically anyone, besides you."

I thought I was good. I have never, ever been asked to write for anything before. I knew there was no way that suddenly, out of the blue, someone was going to ask me to write.

Two mornings later, I woke up to a message from Alison, the friend that Greg had suggested I talk to. She was asking me if I would consider writing a letter for inclusion in a book that she was working on. And no, Greg had not told her a thing.

Shocked.

Stunned.

There isn't a strong enough word for how I felt.

And the worst part was that now I *had* to say yes. Man, God is so sneaky.

But why? Why would God ask *me*? What did He even want me to write about? I was so unbelievably unqualified. So inexperienced. How was I supposed to find an editor? How do you even get a book published? How do I even save stuff I write without losing it? I lose stuff all the time! What does this cost? *We don't have any extra money for this, God!* I simply didn't have the brainpower to figure it all out.

And then He showed me what He wanted me to write about and I panicked even more. I didn't have the emotional energy to work through all the mess that was jumbled inside my head. In the past, every time I'd ever posted anything on Facebook or a blog, I always regretted it because of the vulnerability. I felt so naked; so exposed.

Heck, it took me forever to even refer to myself as having an illness because it made me feel like such a drama queen. I don't know why. It doesn't make sense. But so much about me doesn't make sense.

So why me? Could I really bare my soul to the world? How could I handle being in public after publishing something so personal, always wondering who knew the intimate details of my life?

Every way I looked at it, it was just too much. He was asking *too* much.

Couldn't He see that I simply didn't have it to give? It was a ridiculous request.

Have you ever noticed that the Bible is full of ridiculous requests? Think about the widow of Zarephath from 1 Kings 17. I think that Elijah's request for her to give him food goes down as one of the worst requests in all the Bible.

I mean, seriously. They are in the middle of a drought, with no food in sight *anywhere*. The widow tells Elijah that she only has enough food for one more meal for herself and her son, and then they must die!

I would think that Elijah would have fallen all over himself apologizing. "I'm so sorry. I didn't realize. Oh, of course, forgive me. Your son needs that food."

But instead, the man of God responds, "No biggie. Go ahead and make me some food first."

I think I may have told him just where he could put his walking stick.

I mean, let's see some righteous mama bear rage. *This is my son! It's all we have. You've got some serious nerve trying to convince me to hand over his last meal.*

I can't imagine what this mom was going through. She has already endured unspeakable heartache as she watched her child lose his father. She is all alone, with nothing. No husband, no job, no resources. They are in the middle of a drought, and she has absolutely no way to provide for her son. What was it like to watch their oil and flour dwindle, to eat too little each day and go to bed hungry in an effort to make it last? To watch the sky and hope against hope that rain would come before it was too late?

And still, on that day, she knew that it wasn't enough. She didn't have enough. *She* wasn't enough to save her son.

Have you ever felt like you aren't enough?

You are stretched too thin with too few resources. You don't have the energy or strength for everything that you need to accomplish. You don't have the wisdom to know how to solve all the problems that are urgently pressing before you, and you feel like you have come to the end of yourself.

That is an awful place to be. At the end of yourself. When you are at the end of yourself, and you look ahead, all you see is the pain and that you have zero ability to fix any of it. You can't see a solution. You can't see that it will get any better. But it is also a truly beautiful place to be, because all you see is utter darkness.

And Jesus shines brightest in the dark.

I'm not sure if that is what made the widow say yes to Elijah. Perhaps, she figured she didn't have anything to lose except a few more hours of life. They were going to die anyway, so why not take a chance on this stranger and his foolish suggestion that if she gave all she had when she came to the end of her resources, God would provide.

Whatever her reason, it was a daring move.

Sometimes, when we are at the end of ourselves with no other options, we still want to grasp and grope in the darkness for something. Anything. When we fall at the feet of Jesus and trust that He will provide, even with no other options, it sometimes still feels like a daring move. It seems like a risk.

Until He provides. And you realize that He was worth the risk all along. And not only was He worth the risk, but He was also worth the pain and heartache that led you to the end of yourself in the first place.

Because, dear friend, contrary to what you and I have likely been told our entire lives, we were never, ever, meant to be enough on our own. Only Jesus is. We will always fall short. We will always mess up, and we will always let our families and ourselves down.

But Jesus won't.

Stop trying to fill holes that you were never meant to fill. Stop trying to fill voids that were never meant for you to fill. Your children, your friends, your family, yourself; you all have needs that were only meant to be filled by Jesus. When you ache because your children ache, remember that they aren't supposed to be enough on their own either. Their hardships will also bring them to the only One who can fill them completely. Comfort them, pray with them, and bring them to Jesus so *He* can fill them.

Learning to let Jesus be enough because we are not isn't picture-perfect. In fact, it can be pretty darn ugly, and it is far from easy. It may take many sleepless nights or even years.

But, it will be worth it.

"Therefore let those who suffer according to God's will entrust their souls to a faithful Creator while doing good."

– 1 Peter 4:19, ESV

The widow wasn't enough to save her son. She couldn't meet his needs. But God.

We are not enough, but God is.

The widow made food for Elijah *first* as God was asking of her, and sure enough, every day there was sufficient flour and oil for the day until the rain came.

You are not enough. You can't meet everyone's needs. But that's okay. All you really need is to put God first, as He is asking of you, and *He* will be enough for each day until the Son comes.

Throughout this POTS journey, I have been forced to see my inadequacy in so many ways. I was never—nor will I ever be—capable of dealing with any of it on my own. I felt like I'd lived for years at the end of myself, which was actually right where He wanted me at the time.

Now, I knew I wasn't adequate for this new challenge. I wasn't enough to make this book a reality: not enough experience, energy, strength, finances, skill, or faith. I was lacking in *everything* I needed. But gradually God helped me realize that all my "not enough's" were exactly why He wanted *me*. It is evident through the disciples He chose that He likes to use screwups. And my lack, my obvious inability and my heartache are what will make His glory shine all the brighter because it is painfully obvious that this book didn't come from my own skills and knowledge.

He has already led me in such a mighty way, and it has left me utterly astounded. He only shows me one little step at a time; probably because He knows that if I knew the entire picture from the beginning that I'd run for the hills. But He reveals only as much as I need, and simply equips me for the task set before me.

I don't yet know fully what He has planned. But I do know that all the work is already worth it, because **you are reading this for a reason**, and I know that God has worked in my heart through writing this.

You and me. We are certainly enough to make all the work of creating this book worth it.

I have been stretched and stressed and grown through both illness and writing. I'm confident that God has more for me that He prepared "beforehand." There are things that He has for me not *in spite* of my illness, but *because* of it.

The same is true for you. There are things that you have endured in your life. Perhaps you are enduring them now. But whatever they are, whenever they happened, God wants to redeem them. He is the redeemer of you *and* your life experiences.

So, are you ready? Are you ready to risk looking for Jesus in the depths of your suffering? Are you ready to recognize that He specializes in dwelling within our worst nightmares because His light shines the brightest in the midst of darkness? And perhaps the most difficult question of all ... are you ready to embrace that darkness knowing that it provides you with the greatest means to display His glory?

Even if you answer with a resounding yes, tomorrow, you may not be so sure. It's a process. It's a daily decision to say, "I choose to believe that God's word is true and He works all things together for my good."

> "And we know that all things work together for good to them that love God, to them who are the called according to his purpose."
>
> – Romans 8:28, KJV

All things.

Not some. Not the happy things. Not the fun things.

All things.

God has prepared good works for *you* beforehand knowing what *you* would endure. How can you allow Him to transform your trials into a force for good? It may not happen when the heartache is fresh. God doesn't expect us to ignore our grief. He wants to process it with us. And that takes time.

It takes time because we grow in our trials slowly, much like our muscles. Muscles don't grow when keeping the status quo. They must be stressed. They must be pushed beyond the limits of what they are used to dealing with. There must be greater tension than they are comfortable with; a disruption in their homeostasis. They must, in fact, be damaged. It is localized damage, but damage nonetheless.

Then the body repairs itself by fusing muscle fibers together to form new muscle protein strands or myofibrils. The myofibrils increase in thickness and quantity, resulting in hypertrophy.

But here is the kicker: you don't see the growth during the period of stress. Your muscles don't grow during your workout. The workout sucks! Those myofibrils don't do their thing till later on.

The growth occurs while you rest.

This is often the case with the stress we experience. Anxiety, broken relationships and suffering can leave us feeling pretty damaged. But if we never rest and we never stop to listen; if we are constantly rushing from one crisis to the next, trying to bail water from the boat, then there is no time for the growth to occur. Sometimes we need to stop to simply see a hole that could be filled to prevent the water from seeping in the boat in the first place.

Other times, there is no solution to be found. The issue is much more complex and all-encompassing. But we cannot process our emotions and begin to grow from these experiences without taking the time to step back and take it all in. To ponder, rest, pray and listen. To allow God to begin to whisper clues as to how He wants to use your pain to draw you to Him and what greater good can result from it.

From a very young age, we are taught the six big questions to ask. Who, what, where, when, why and how. In most of our life circumstances, it's pretty obvious what happened, where it happened, when it happened and who it involved. But the question of *why* it happened ... that is where we get stuck. It's natural to want to know why. Why did I get POTS? Why do my children struggle with their own health issues? Why did I have miscarriages?

You have your own "whys." Why did my spouse leave me? Why didn't I have a stable family as a child? Why can't I get back on my feet? Why did my child have to get sick? I'm sure you have a lot of whys.

Sometimes we cruise along in life and only give our whys a passing thought. Other times, our whys eat us alive, literally stealing our very breath. The tricky thing about real life whys—the thing that you aren't taught when asking those six big questions in school as a child—is that usually, there is no answer to be found. At least not on this side of eternity.

Still, we ask. And we ask. And we ask. We are stuck with no answer, bitter because we can't finish the assignment and move on to another subject. Sometimes, the bell has rung, and life is passing us by. And we forget. We forget that we were supposed to eventually move past the five Ws.

We forget that there is a sixth question that we are supposed to ask, because we never got past the fifth.

How?

How. It's a tiny word, much like why. But I find that while why has an incredible power for negativity, how has unlimited power for pulling us out of the mud. Why is a breeding ground for resentment, bitterness and pity parties. How is the first step to viewing your worst life experiences as a force for good.

How can I learn from this?

How does my story fit into God's grand narrative?

How can this bring me closer to God?

How can I use my hard experiences to help others?

And perhaps the questions that did the most to pull me out of the muck that illness had sunk me into: how could I let my suffering go to waste? How can I live with this if I don't allow God to recycle it for good?

So, where are you, dear friend? What whys have you been asking? Was your big dream worldwide missions too, and you're asking why it was taken away? Maybe. Maybe your big dream was the perfect family that included a husband with a great job that allowed you to stay home with your 2.5 kids. Maybe that dream was shattered by the devastating pain of divorce. Your dream may seem like it is gone forever, and life is painstakingly hard. Time is short and moments of happiness are small, and you want to know why this has happened to you.

Maybe your big dream was a big family. The pitter-patter of many feet. The squeals and squabbles. You were ready for it all. But after your first, infertility left your baby as an only child. You are so incredibly grateful for the precious soul God gave you, but this is not what you wanted for you or for her. And you want to know the answer to the burning question: why didn't God allow you to have more?

I don't know where you are on your journey. This old world offers far too many heartaches for me to guess. I could never tell you why your pain happened. But I can guarantee you this: if you sincerely ask God how He wants to recycle your heartache, He will always bring growth and beauty out of your painful, small or mundane life.

Actually, He can do that more powerfully through a difficult life than He can through an easy one. But you must look for Him to do it. And that starts by letting go of why and embracing how.

You must look for *how* His glory can be shown. Not *in spite of* your broken dream, but *because* your dream has been cut down to size. Your growth and His glory go hand in hand. And your growth does not happen when everything is sunshine and roses.

When things are going great, we don't look to change anything. So, there isn't much chance for growth. But when things are bad? In fact, the worse things get, the more likely we are to make a change. Even if it's just a change of perspective, that's growth, and sometimes that's enough to make all the difference in the world.

There are times when I desperately want to be made physically whole again. I hear friends tell stories of taking their kids camping or going on amazing hikes and I salivate. That longing is still there. That jealousy and yes, sometimes even resentment rears its ugly head. Sometimes I think I would give almost anything to be able to do those things again; to be able to go to a ball game in the heat without running through my POTS safety checklist. I would love for my kids to have a taste of their mother that existed before POTS entered our world. But those are all things that I want *some* of the time.

Do you know what I want *all* of the time? To live the life God has for me. To learn the things that He wants me to know, to be the person who He wants me to be. To serve in the capacity that He wants me to serve. If I have those things, then circumstances do not determine the level of joy in my life.

Does all of this sound like all pain can be wrapped up with a lovely little bow; that there is a sexy side to suffering? We all know that is not true. There is beauty. There is reward. There is gain. But in the midst of it, it downright sucks. It ain't pretty. And let's face it, some trials will not have an end till Jesus wipes them all out.

However, I was more than willing to give up time, money and energy to serve in mission work. We are all willing to make sacrifices for the things that we see value in. I just needed to learn the value of the things that I didn't fully know. Call me crazy, but I think taking on challenges—even big ones like chronic illness—in this temporary life in order to gain a new perspective and understanding of what it means to know the God who is eternal, is a fair trade. No, it's better than that.

It's a trade *up*.

I'd like not to have POTS. But given the choice to go back and do it all again without it, I don't think I'd make that choice. I wouldn't be the person I am without my health conditions. I wouldn't know God like I do without it.

What about you?

If you could go back, would you give up your heartache? Would you let go of the lessons and blessings that God is trying to teach you through it? Would you be willing to sacrifice the things that God wants to do in your life *because* of your pain? Or can you embrace the knowledge that you are, in light of eternity, better when you're broken? Can you begin to see your heartache as a blessing in disguise?

I know. It's such an incredible disguise that it's nearly impossible to recognize it for what it truly is. And it's such a hard step to take. That step where you begin to bridge the gap between grief and anger and wishing it away and asking why to choosing to believe that this heartache is for your good. That step where you move closer to being able to see how God is going to use this for good.

Let's face it; it's not a stable bridge. It's made of ropes and rotten boards, and it swings wildly with every gust of wind the devil sends your way. It is high over the gorge of losses, misunderstandings, judgment and pride. Each step is frightening. Sometimes the boards creak and you think they will break, so you take a few steps backward. You look down to regain your footing and see what others are thinking of you and retreat further back toward your own grief.

But through your sorrow He continues to call you, so you look up to the other side. You realize that if you keep your eyes on Him, you don't see what others are thinking. You don't see how fragile the bridge is. You simply don't focus on all the loss. And by looking to Him, you are slowly able to put one foot in front of the other and make progress across the bridge.

That journey is a frightening one to embark on, and you will doubt yourself at times, but it is the most freeing journey you will ever take.

And it is most definitely a trade up.

What do you say? Will you take that journey with me?

It won't be easy, but it will be worth it.

P.S.

When you wake up tomorrow morning, don't forget to focus on Him and take another step.

And I promise to do the same right along with you.

ACKNOWLEDGMENTS

To Bryan and Deedee Heathman at Made for Success Publishing, thank you for believing in the message of this book and for opening your home and hearts to me. God poured belief into me through you.

Katie Rios, you were God's unexpected cherry on top. An editor who knows my struggles so intimately was beyond my wildest dreams. Thank you for your countless hours combing through the jumbled mess pouring from my mind.

My cousins, Joanne and Peyton, thank you for your enthusiasm and the beautiful pictures you created of our family and the somewhat decent picture of me. You are the best.

Thank you to so many friends, Jade, Lacey, Angel and many others who asked questions, gave advice, prayed and encouraged along the way.

My siblings, Wendi, Kimi, Travis and Kristen, throughout this entire process, your words of encouragement and feedback on the manuscript have meant so much. My sibs rock!

My in-laws, the best a girl could ask for, Sandy, Kip and Melissa. Your excitement and immediate enthusiasm helped give me the courage to pursue this goal. Thank you for your continued support from start to end.

My grandpa, "Ganggang" who was thrilled that I was writing this book but passed away just before it was completed. Ganggang never needed words to teach me the freedom of trusting God with the difficult and how to attempt things beyond my means with a wild, crazy expectancy—giddy to see how God will come through. He was the finest example of Christ and his legacy lives on, inspires and glorifies the God he loved so dearly.

My grandma, "Bobane" your excitement to read the manuscript and the way you tore through it brought a smile to my heart and courage to allow others to read. Your courage and faith in the face of such loss is an inspiration.

Mom and Dad, without you instilling a steadfast faith in what God can do, I would never have had the courage to attempt writing this book. Your excitement from the start and belief in me mean the world. Thank you for all your help from watching the kids while I visited my publisher to understanding the lack of help I was able to give the family while working on this project. I am so blessed to have you.

Aiden, Noah and Carrington, thank you for being the light of my life. Your laughter is the most beautiful sound on earth and each of you teach me new things every day. Your excitement, hundreds of questions and desire to share our story have encouraged me more than you could know. Thank you for understanding and being willing to sacrifice time with me while I was stuck behind a computer screen. Seeing you grow to love Jesus brings me more joy than anything else in this world. You are each made for a great purpose and I pray that you will stay close to God and that He would use you to enlarge His kingdom. I am so proud of each of you and love you more than words can express.

Greg, none of this would have happened without you. Your undying support and belief in me and in God's ability to come through help drive me on. Thank you for taking on so many roles you never signed up for. Thank you for being willing to be vulnerable along with me. Thank you for loving me so well. I love you.

"My precious Jesus, because your love is better than life, my lips will glorify you ..." (Psalm 63:3) even when You make me do terrifying things like write a book. What's happening in my life doesn't change the incredibleness of Your love. So I praise You. And I love You. Because of You I *always* have a reason to smile and give thanks.

LETTER TO CAREGIVERS

What We Wish Our Friends and Family Knew

A letter to those who have supported us, and those who wish they could but don't know how

It may seem obvious, but we do not want to be sick. We already feel like complete drama queens (or kings) at times, and are embarrassed that everything involving us can be exasperatingly complicated ... so we desperately need your support. More than anything else, we need you to *believe us*. You cannot see our illness—often because we do our best to look like everyone else. But that doesn't mean it isn't there. All. The. Time.

You may see us out smiling and laughing, occasionally even standing for long periods of time. Don't assume that we are suddenly well or that we have been faking an illness on the days we can't even sit upright. Sometimes we may be feeling better than usual (often for no logical reason). Or, we could be pushing ourselves harder than you could ever imagine, and you can't tell because we've become experts at playing our part in the chronic illness social play.

In this play, although we have the lead role, we feel more like the lights and camera guy—no one sees what we really do. No one knows the lengths we go to in order to pull this production off.

Why are we so fake, you ask? It's not that we are being fake. It's that sometimes, we just want to be normal like everyone else. And we feel like if we are not normal at times, then everyone will become even more sick of our story than we are. We want to talk and laugh and enjoy being with other people. And sadly, that requires hiding what is truly happening inside.

We can be completely fine one minute and a hot mess the next. And vice versa. We completely understand how it could appear that our symptoms are questionable. But, we can assure you that they are very real, and we like the unpredictability even less than you do. We need you to believe us.

We also want to be productive, and the very last thing we want is to be a burden. We work as hard as our bodies will allow, and usually harder than we should. If we have a good day, we typically overdo it by trying to catch up on everything we've missed. However, the price we pay for overdoing it is something that isn't seen by most. If we are out having a good time because it's a better-than-usual day, we will likely be recovering for the next day (or several).

You might hear us talk about "using too many spoons." This is when we've used up all the energy in our reservoir and have to lay low to refill. We traveled too many miles in order to socialize or work, and we are paying for it, whether you see it or not. Christine Miserandio first introduced this concept as the "spoon theory," giving language to the daily struggles of chronic illness sufferers.[1]

A normal young healthy person has a virtually unlimited number of "spoons." Their limitation tends to be how many

---

[1] Miserandio, Christine. The Spoon Theory. https://butyoudontlooksick.com/articles/written-by-christine/the-spoon-theory/

hours there are in a day rather than energy to accomplish their tasks. They can get dressed, take a shower, make a meal and do laundry without even thinking about it. Those of us that battle a chronic illness will have to ration our energy depending on how many "spoons" we woke up with that day. Wake up with only three spoons? Today you have the choice to either shower or stand to cook a meal.

Seemingly simple tasks take an extraordinary amount of energy, and we have very little to begin with. When we invite you over and take time to socialize, it is a sacrifice that we may likely pay for over the next couple days. Please know that doesn't mean we don't want to socialize or be around people; it just means we have to be very strategic with the way we live our lives. You know we really love you when we want to be around you on a low spoon day! And we hope that you know that we still love you even when we simply can't be around.

Our fear, now that you understand our "spoon limited life," is that you will not ask us to go out or attend events anymore. We don't want you thinking, *Well, she can't use up her spoons by going to dinner with me.* Although it is possible that we won't have the energy available for dinner or that we may need to conserve the energy we have for other responsibilities, the invitation still means so much. We still long to be included.

We also need you to support us in our search for answers. It can be a long journey to a diagnosis, and we can start to doubt ourselves along the way. Please believe in us and let us know that we are worth the time, energy and money it takes to find the answer.

Sometimes we don't know how to ask for help, or we are too embarrassed. We don't want to burden those we love the most. When you can, jump in and do something that you know is a struggle for us. Make a meal and bring it over, offer to help with cleaning, watch the kids, or just come over and remind us we aren't alone. It means the world to be supported in this way.

We also want you to still be able to enjoy your life. We want you to hike, run, camp, take a shower standing up and do anything active that you love to do—even if we can't. But we want you to appreciate it. We want you to think about what you are doing, and to see your abilities for the gifts and blessings that they are.

Lastly, if you don't know what to do, just say so. Don't try to expound on an experience that you haven't faced yourself; just say that you don't understand, but you are there for us anyway. Ask us to tell you what it's like to live a day in our shoes. We won't be able to completely explain it. But we often feel isolated, and although we don't want to feel like we are boring everyone with our depressing story, we also have a deep need for those we love to have some small insight into our world.

You are such an important part of our lives, so draw near and let us know that although illness may have changed our world, it hasn't changed your love for us.

Because it certainly has not changed our love for you.

Thank you for all the big and little things that you do for us. They do not go unnoticed.

Appendix

Okay, I can't include a medical resource without the obligatory cover-my-hinny info. I must admit this feels akin to the sticker on your blow dryer that says, "Do not use while showering." But alas, it must be stated.

So here goes: This is by no means a comprehensive list of treatments and tests available. In fact, it is likely quite limited, but it is the best that Greg and I could come up with together without ending up, um ... not together. All patients are different and have different needs. Each one will need to work with their doctor to find the right combination of treatments that work for them. Please do not construe any information in this resource as personal medical advice.

Mmmkay?

You may proceed.

Appendix A:
Treatment Overview

Non-pharmacologic Treatments

Treatment	Mechanism of Action/ Benefits	Adverse Reactions and limitations
Exercise	Expands blood volume, reconditions muscles, improves venous return	Exacerbation of symptoms, it sucks
Oral Hydration	Expands blood volume	Hyponatremia (low blood sodium)
Electrolyte Drinks	Adds salts so you retain fluid and keep blood pressure up	High volume of sugar and additives
Salt Supplementation	Expands blood volume	Difficult without salt tablets
Cooling Vests	Helps regulate temperature in the heat and avoid excessive vasodilation	Inconvenience of keeping vest cool during transport, may appear that you are packing a bomb
Compression Stockings	Enhances venous return, slimming, instant butt lift	Discomfort, difficult to put on and take off, hot in the summer
IV 0.9% sodium chloride solution infusions	Expands blood volume	Access complications and inconvenience
Prebiotics	Feeds good bacteria so it flourishes	Symptoms of detox are possible with high-quality prebiotics
Probiotics	Adds good bacteria, helps balance normal flora, improves gut health, decreases inflammation	Temporary symptoms of detox possible: rashes, headache, nausea, fatigue

Pharmacologic Treatments

Treatment	Mechanism of action/ Benefits	Adverse reactions and limitations
Fludrocortisone	Expands blood volume	Swelling of the legs and low potassium
Desmopressin	Expands blood volume	Low blood sodium
Propranolol	Reduces tachycardia/ palpitations	Low blood pressure, fatigue, symptom exacerbation
Midodrine	Enhances venous return; reduces tachycardia	Headache, scalp tingling, hair standing up (piloerection)
Pyridostigmine	Enhances venous return; reduces tachycardia	Diarrhea
Clonidine	Reduces tachycardia	Mental clouding, fatigue, peripheral vasodilatation
Ivabradine	Reduces tachycardia	Headaches, bradycardia
H1 and H2 Antagonists	Blocks histamine action	Drowsiness
Cromolyn Sodium	Decreases histamine release	Rash
Aspirin	Blocks histamine action	Gastrointestinal upset and bleeding
Sudafed	Vasoconstriction	Tachycardia, insomnia, elevated blood pressure
Octreotide	Systemic vasoconstriction; helps low blood pressure after eating	Abdominal pain and diarrhea Injection only
Methylphenidate	Vasoconstriction	Decreased appetite, insomnia, abdominal pain
Bupropion	Keeps norepinephrine (vasoconstrictor) and dopamine circulating, blocks inflammatory mediators, decreases neuropathic pain	Decreases appetite, hypertension, increased risk of seizures with sudden withdrawal
Erythropoietin	Stimulates red cell growth to increase the number of red blood cells and central volume	Expensive, low efficacy in studies so often a last resort

The above extrapolated from: *Journal of the American Academy of PAs 29(4):17-23, April 2016* and *Journal of Arrhythmia Vol 27 No 4 2011, Mizumaki, Koichi MD PhD pages 289-306*

Appendix B:
Diagnostic Test Overview

Cardiac Testing

Tilt Table Test: Way to find the cause of syncope or pre-syncope (dizziness and lightheadedness) and see if it is related to the heart output and gravity. The patient lies on a bed and is tilted up to 75 degrees. Machines monitor your blood pressure, heart rate, EKG and oxygen levels to watch for changes with position. Also, a way to be diagnosed as an alien or irritate highly respected electrophysiologists.

Stress Test: Test of cardiovascular capacity made by monitoring the heart rate during a period of increasingly strenuous exercise, this can be done with Echocardiogram or without. It can also be chemically induced (using medication to make the heart rate increase). **WARNING**: May induce feelings of aggression and anger if the recommended treatment is "more exercise."

Echocardiogram: Using an ultrasound machine to take a standard two-dimensional, three-dimensional and Doppler ultrasound to create images of the heart.

Electrocardiogram (EKG or ECG): Simple, short picture of electrical activity of the heart from different angles.

Electrophysiology (EP) study: Used to diagnose abnormal heartbeats or arrhythmia. The test is performed by inserting catheters—followed by wire electrodes—through blood vessels that enter the heart to measure electrical activity. This is usually only done if there is suspicion of damage to the electrical system of the heart.

Holter Monitor: 1-2 day monitor to evaluate the EKG rhythm of the heart, watching for abnormal beats or arrhythmias that may cause symptoms.

30-day Event Monitor: 30-day monitor to evaluate the EKG rhythm of the heart watching for abnormal beats or arrhythmias that may cause symptoms. And if you've been dying to gain weight, you're in luck. The monitor instantly adds two inches to your waist for a full 30 days.

Implantable Cardiac Monitor: 2-5-year implanted monitor to evaluate the EKG rhythm of the heart, watching for abnormal beats or arrhythmias that may cause symptoms.

Advanced Imaging

CAT Scan (Computerized Axial Tomography): Specialized X-ray study that uses computers to see structures in the body.

CTA Scan (Computerized Tomography Angiogram): Specialized X-ray study that uses computers to see specific blood vessels and look for abnormalities. This test WILL make you think you've peed your pants, so don't panic. (Although, I did anyway.)

MRI (Magnetic Resonance Imaging): Specialized imaging study that uses magnetic fields to see specific structures of the body. No radiation is used. This is better to see soft tissues than a CAT scan and can help see abnormalities with multiple sclerosis and other inflammatory conditions. It is also more sensitive for finding stroke damage. People with medical implants that have ferrite or electronics may be excluded from this test due to the strong magnet used. If you are claustrophobic, you will want to ask for an open MRI or at the very least some seriously strong happy-meds.

MRA (Magnetic Resonance Angiography): Specialized imaging study of the blood vessels using an MRI machine.

Specialized Neurologic Testing

EMG (Electro Myelogram): This is a test that checks the conductivity of the peripheral nervous system. It uses needles to send electrical current through muscles and nerves to check for impedance issues (breaks in the line). It can test for poor conduction and neuropathy (large fiber). This test can be painful for some patients, due to the electrical current used (like an electrical shock). Side effects may include feelings of frustration and anxiety if the resulting diagnosis is "just anxiety."

Small Fiber Neuropathy Biopsy: A biopsy taking a plug of skin (punch biopsy) can test for damage to the nervous system. It looks for the density of small fibers under the microscope. In general, small fiber neuropathy cannot be picked up on an EMG test due to the limitations of the EMG.

Appendix C:
Different Paths for Diagnosis and Treatment

Conventional Medicine: This is the current mainstream medical diagnosis, treatment, and prevention of diseases by use of drugs, radiation, and surgery. It is coordinated by *medical* doctors (MD or DO trained physicians) and other healthcare professionals. The goal is to restore health by the prevention and treatment of illness. This is what we know as modern medicine.

Naturopathic Medicine: Uses both nature and modern science. Naturopathic medicine focuses on holistic, proactive prevention and comprehensive diagnosis and treatment. Common focuses are on diet, lifestyle modifications and detoxification to assist the body in healing itself. Often, symptom suppression is avoided if possible.

Due to a lack of licensure standards in many states, there can be a wide array of skill sets and knowledge levels.

Integrative Medicine: Conventional medicine integrated with nonconventional or alternative modalities and naturopathy. It may or may not be focused on the root cause of illness.

Functional Medicine: Similar to integrative medicine; however, prevention and management of the root cause of disease is always the focus. This is the medical practice or treatments that focus on optimal functioning of the body and its organs, usually involving systems of holistic or alternative medicine as well as traditional and natural medicine.

Resources

http://www.dysautonomiainternational.org has a ton of helpful information on all the conditions under the dysautonomia umbrella, as well as other articles, patient stories, awareness and events. This is a great place to start if you've just been diagnosed, or suspect you have one of these conditions.

The Journal of the American Academy of Physician Assistants has an incredibly informative article detailing evaluation, symptoms, diagnosis and treatment of POTS on their website. Head over to https://journals.lww.com/jaapa, and search for the article titled **"Recognizing postural orthostatic tachycardia syndrome."**

About Author

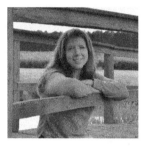

C risty Maddox is an author and mother of three who loves Jesus. She and her BFF, Greg have been married for 20 years. A true love for God was birthed through her chronic illness. Cristy has a passion for helping others find the hidden gems He has waiting for them in their broken dreams. Cristy loves people, but is a homebody who writes from her kitchen table in the middle of rural Virginia.

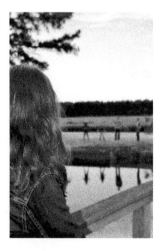